Advanced Probability Theory for Biomedical Engineers

Copyright © 2006 by Morgan & Claypool

All rights reserved. No part of this publication may be reproduced, stored in a retrieval system, or transmitted in any form or by any means—electronic, mechanical, photocopy, recording, or any other except for brief quotations in printed reviews, without the prior permission of the publisher.

Advanced Probability Theory for Biomedical Engineers
John D. Enderle, David C. Farden, and Daniel J. Krause
www.morganclaypool.com

ISBN-10: 1598291505   paperback
ISBN-13: 9781598291506   paperback

ISBN-10: 1598291513   ebook
ISBN-13: 9781598291513   ebook

DOI 10.2200/S00063ED1V01Y200610BME011

A lecture in the Morgan & Claypool Synthesis Series
SYNTHESIS LECTURES ON BIOMEDICAL ENGINEERING #11

Lecture #11
Series Editor: John D. Enderle, University of Connecticut

Series ISSN: 1930-0328   print

Series ISSN: 1930-0336   electronic

First Edition
10 9 8 7 6 5 4 3 2 1

Printed in the United States of America

Advanced Probability Theory for Biomedical Engineers

John D. Enderle
Program Director & Professor for Biomedical Engineering,
University of Connecticut

David C. Farden
Professor of Electrical and Computer Engineering,
North Dakota State University

Daniel J. Krause
Emeritus Professor of Electrical and Computer Engineering,
North Dakota State University

SYNTHESIS LECTURES ON BIOMEDICAL ENGINEERING #11

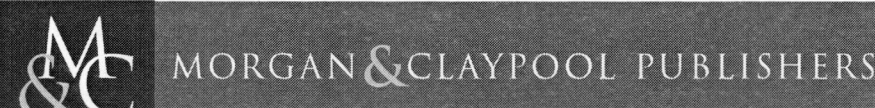

ABSTRACT

This is the third in a series of short books on probability theory and random processes for biomedical engineers. This book focuses on standard probability distributions commonly encountered in biomedical engineering. The exponential, Poisson and Gaussian distributions are introduced, as well as important approximations to the Bernoulli PMF and Gaussian CDF. Many important properties of jointly Gaussian random variables are presented. The primary subjects of the final chapter are methods for determining the probability distribution of a function of a random variable. We first evaluate the probability distribution of a function of one random variable using the CDF and then the PDF. Next, the probability distribution for a single random variable is determined from a function of two random variables using the CDF. Then, the joint probability distribution is found from a function of two random variables using the joint PDF and the CDF.

The aim of all three books is as an introduction to probability theory. The audience includes students, engineers and researchers presenting applications of this theory to a wide variety of problems—as well as pursuing these topics at a more advanced level. The theory material is presented in a logical manner—developing special mathematical skills as needed. The mathematical background required of the reader is basic knowledge of differential calculus. Pertinent biomedical engineering examples are throughout the text. Drill problems, straightforward exercises designed to reinforce concepts and develop problem solution skills, follow most sections.

KEYWORDS

Probability Theory, Random Processes, Engineering Statistics, Probability and Statistics for Biomedical Engineers, Exponential distributions, Poisson distributions, Gaussian distributions Bernoulli PMF and Gaussian CDF. Gaussian random variables

Contents

5. **Standard Probability Distributions** 1
   5.1 Uniform Distributions 1
   5.2 Exponential Distributions 4
   5.3 Bernoulli Trials 6
       5.3.1 Poisson Approximation to Bernoulli 11
       5.3.2 Gaussian Approximation to Bernoulli 12
   5.4 Poisson Distribution 14
       5.4.1 Interarrival Times 18
   5.5 Univariate Gaussian Distribution 20
       5.5.1 Marcum's Q Function 25
   5.6 Bivariate Gaussian Random Variables 26
       5.6.1 Constant Contours 32
   5.7 Summary 36
   5.8 Problems 36

6. **Transformations of Random Variables** 45
   6.1 Univariate CDF Technique 45
       6.1.1 CDF Technique with Monotonic Functions 45
       6.1.2 CDF Technique with Arbitrary Functions 46
   6.2 Univariate PDF Technique 53
       6.2.1 Continuous Random Variable 53
       6.2.2 Mixed Random Variable 56
       6.2.3 Conditional PDF Technique 57
   6.3 One Function of Two Random Variables 59
   6.4 Bivariate Transformations 63
       6.4.1 Bivariate CDF Technique 63
       6.4.2 Bivariate PDF Technique 65
   6.5 Summary 73
   6.6 Problems 75

Preface

This is the third in a series of short books on probability theory and random processes for biomedical engineers. This text is written as an introduction to probability theory. The goal was to prepare students at the sophomore, junior or senior level for the application of this theory to a wide variety of problems - as well as pursue these topics at a more advanced level. Our approach is to present a unified treatment of the subject. There are only a few key concepts involved in the basic theory of probability theory. These key concepts are all presented in the first chapter. The second chapter introduces the topic of random variables. The third chapter focuses on expectation, standard deviation, moments, and the characteristic function. In addition, conditional expectation, conditional moments and the conditional characteristic function are also discussed. The fourth chapter introduces jointly distributed random variables, along with joint expectation, joint moments, and the joint characteristic function. Convolution is also developed. Later chapters simply expand upon these key ideas and extend the range of application.

This short book focuses on standard probability distributions commonly encountered in biomedical engineering. Here in Chapter 5, the exponential, Poisson and Gaussian distributions are introduced, as well as important approximations to the Bernoulli PMF and Gaussian CDF. Many important properties of *jointly* distributed Gaussian random variables are presented. The primary subjects of Chapter 6 are methods for determining the probability distribution of a function of a random variable. We first evaluate the probability distribution of a function of one random variable using the CDF and then the PDF. Next, the probability distribution for a single random variable is determined from a function of two random variables using the CDF. Then, the joint probability distribution is found from a function of two random variables using the joint PDF and the CDF.

A considerable effort has been made to develop the theory in a logical manner - developing special mathematical skills as needed. The mathematical background required of the reader is basic knowledge of differential calculus. Every effort has been made to be consistent with commonly used notation and terminology—both within the engineering community as well as the probability and statistics literature.

The applications and examples given reflect the authors' background in teaching probability theory and random processes for many years. We have found it best to introduce this material using simple examples such as dice and cards, rather than more complex biological and biomedical phenomena. However, we do introduce some pertinent biomedical engineering examples throughout the text.

Students in other fields should also find the approach useful. Drill problems, straightforward exercises designed to reinforce concepts and develop problem solution skills, follow most sections. The answers to the drill problems follow the problem statement in random order. At the end of each chapter is a wide selection of problems, ranging from simple to difficult, presented in the same general order as covered in the textbook.

We acknowledge and thank William Pruehsner for the technical illustrations. Many of the examples and end of chapter problems are based on examples from the textbook by Drake [9].

CHAPTER 5

Standard Probability Distributions

A surprisingly small number of probability distributions describe many natural probabilistic phenomena. This chapter presents some of these discrete and continuous probability distributions that occur often enough in a variety of problems to deserve special mention. We will see that many random variables and their corresponding experiments have similar properties and can be described by the same probability distribution. Each section introduces a new PMF or PDF. Following this, the mean, variance, and characteristic function are found. Additionally, special properties are pointed out along with relationships among other probability distributions. In some instances, the PMF or PDF is derived according to the characteristics of the experiment. Because of the vast number of probability distributions, we cannot possibly discuss them all here in this chapter.

5.1 UNIFORM DISTRIBUTIONS

Definition 5.1.1. *The discrete RV x has a **uniform distribution** over n points ($n > 1$) on the interval $[a, b]$ if x is a lattice RV with span $h = (b-a)/(n-1)$ and PMF*

$$p_x(\alpha) = \begin{cases} 1/n, & \alpha = kh + a, k = 0, 1, \ldots, n-1 \\ 0, & \text{otherwise.} \end{cases} \tag{5.1}$$

The mean and variance of a discrete uniform RV are easily computed with the aid of Lemma 2.3.1:

$$\eta_x = \frac{1}{n}\sum_{k=0}^{n-1}(kh+a) = \frac{h}{n}\frac{\gamma_n^{[2]}}{2} + a = \frac{1}{n}\frac{b-a}{n-1}\frac{n(n-1)}{2} + a = \frac{b+a}{2}, \tag{5.2}$$

and

$$\sigma_x^2 = \frac{1}{n}\sum_{k=0}^{n-1}\left(kh - \frac{b-a}{2}\right)^2 = \frac{(b-a)^2}{n}\sum_{k=0}^{n-1}\left(\frac{k^2}{(n-1)^2} - \frac{k}{n-1} + \frac{1}{4}\right). \tag{5.3}$$

Simplifying,

$$\sigma_x^2 = \frac{(b-a)^2}{12}\frac{n+1}{n-1}. \tag{5.4}$$

2 ADVANCED PROBABILITY THEORY FOR BIOMEDICAL ENGINEERS

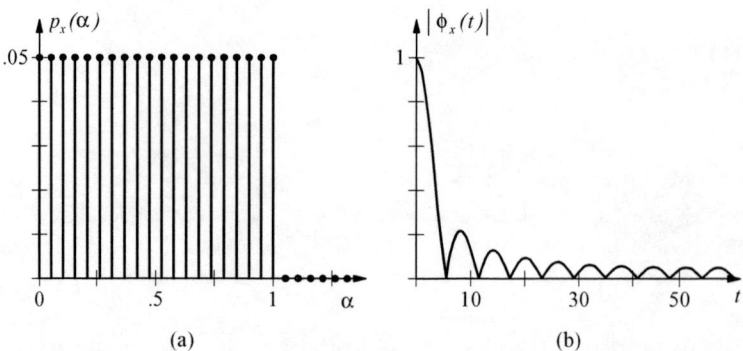

FIGURE 5.1: (a) PMF and (b) characteristic function magnitude for discrete RV with uniform distribution over 20 points on [0, 1].

The characteristic function can be found using the sum of a geometric series:

$$\phi_x(t) = \frac{e^{jat}}{n} \sum_{k=0}^{n-1} (e^{jht})^k = \frac{e^{jat}}{n} \frac{1 - e^{jhnt}}{1 - e^{jht}}. \tag{5.5}$$

Simplifying with the aid of Euler's identity,

$$\phi_x(t) = \exp\left(j\frac{a+b}{2}t\right) \frac{\sin\left(\frac{b-a}{2}\frac{n}{n-1}t\right)}{n \sin\left(\frac{b-a}{2}\frac{1}{n-1}t\right)}. \tag{5.6}$$

Figure 5.1 illustrates the PMF and the magnitude of the characteristic function for a discrete RV which is uniformly distributed over 20 points on [0, 1]. The characteristic function is plotted over $[0, \pi/h]$, where the span $h = 1/19$. Recall from Section 3.3 that $\phi_x(-t) = \phi_x^*(t)$ and that $\phi_x(t)$ is periodic in t with period $2\pi/h$. Thus, Figure 5.1 illustrates one-half period of $|\phi_x(\cdot)|$.

Definition 5.1.2. *The continuous RV x has a **uniform distribution** on the interval $[a, b]$ if x has PDF*

$$f_x(\alpha) = \begin{cases} 1/(b-a), & a \leq \alpha \leq b \\ 0, & \text{otherwise}. \end{cases} \tag{5.7}$$

The mean and variance of a continuous uniform RV are easily computed directly:

$$\eta_x = \frac{1}{b-a} \int_a^b \alpha \, d\alpha = \frac{b^2 - a^2}{2(b-a)} = \frac{b+a}{2}, \tag{5.8}$$

STANDARD PROBABILITY DISTRIBUTIONS 3

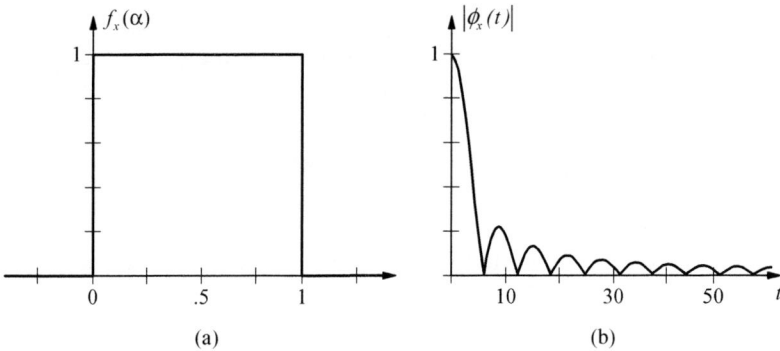

FIGURE 5.2: (a) PDF and (b) characteristic function magnitude for continuous RV with uniform distribution on [0, 1].

and

$$\sigma_x^2 = \frac{1}{b-a} \int_a^b \left(\alpha - \frac{b+a}{2}\right)^2 d\alpha = \frac{(b-a)^2}{12}. \quad (5.9)$$

The characteristic function can be found as

$$\phi_x(t) = \frac{1}{b-a} \int_a^b e^{j\alpha t} d\alpha = \frac{\exp\left(j\frac{b+a}{2}t\right)}{b-a} \int_{-(b-a)/2}^{(b-a)/2} e^{j\alpha t} d\alpha.$$

Simplifying with the aid of Euler's identity,

$$\phi_x(t) = \exp\left(j\frac{a+b}{2}t\right) \frac{\sin\left(\frac{b-a}{2}t\right)}{\frac{b-a}{2}t}. \quad (5.10)$$

Figure 5.2 illustrates the PDF and the magnitude of the characteristic function for a continuous RV uniformly distributed on [0, 1]. Note that the characteristic function in this case is not periodic but $\phi_x(-t) = \phi_x^*(t)$.

Drill Problem 5.1.1. *A pentahedral die (with faces labeled 0,1,2,3,4) is tossed once. Let x be a random variable equaling ten times the number tossed. Determine: (a) p_x (20), (b) $P(10 \leq x \leq 50)$, (c) $E(x)$, (d) σ_x^2.*

Answers: 20, 0.8, 200, 0.2.

Drill Problem 5.1.2. *Random variable x is uniformly distributed on the interval $[-1, 5]$. Determine: (a) F_x (0), (b) $F_x(5)$, (c) η_x, (d) σ_x^2.*

Answers: 1, 1/6, 3, 2.

4 ADVANCED PROBABILITY THEORY FOR BIOMEDICAL ENGINEERS

5.2 EXPONENTIAL DISTRIBUTIONS

Definition 5.2.1. *The discrete RV x has a **geometric distribution** or **discrete exponential distribution** with parameter $p(0 < p < 1)$ if x has PMF*

$$p_x(\alpha) = \begin{cases} p(1-p)^{\alpha-1}, & \alpha = 1, 2, \ldots \\ 0, & \text{otherwise.} \end{cases} \qquad (5.11)$$

The characteristic function can be found using the sum of a geometric series ($q = 1 - p$):

$$\phi_x(t) = \frac{p}{q} \sum_{k=1}^{\infty} \left(q e^{jt}\right)^k = \frac{p e^{jt}}{1 - q e^{jt}}. \qquad (5.12)$$

The mean and variance of a discrete RV with a geometric distribution can be computed using the moment generating property of the characteristic function. The results are

$$\eta_x = \frac{1}{p}, \quad \text{and} \quad \sigma_x^2 = \frac{q}{p^2}. \qquad (5.13)$$

Figure 5.3 illustrates the PMF and the characteristic function magnitude for a discrete RV with geometric distribution and parameter $p = 0.18127$.

It can be shown that a discrete exponentially distributed RV has a memoryless property:

$$p_{x|x>\ell}(\alpha | x > \ell) = p_x(\alpha - \ell), \quad \ell \geq 0. \qquad (5.14)$$

Definition 5.2.2. *The continuous RV x has an **exponential distribution** with parameter $\lambda (\lambda > 0)$ if x has PDF*

$$f_x(\alpha) = \lambda e^{-\lambda \alpha} u(\alpha), \qquad (5.15)$$

where $u(\cdot)$ is the unit step function.

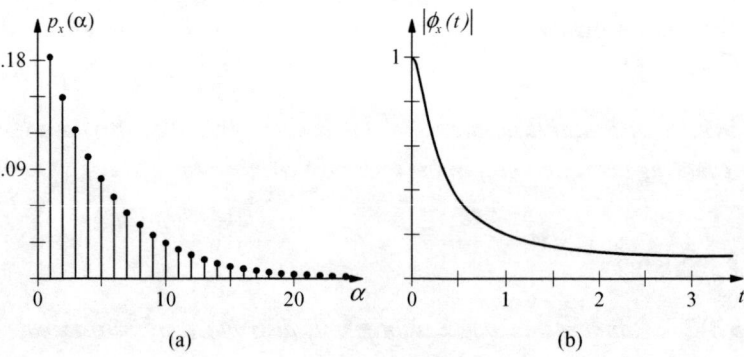

FIGURE 5.3: (a) PMF and (b) characteristic function magnitude for discrete RV with geometric distribution [$p = 0.18127$].

STANDARD PROBABILITY DISTRIBUTIONS 5

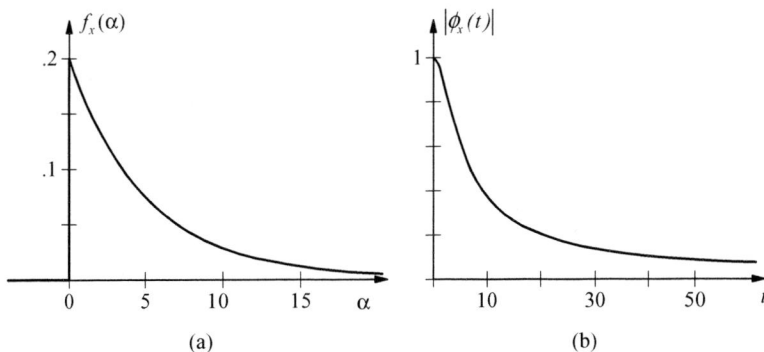

FIGURE 5.4: (a) PDF and (b) characteristic function magnitude for continuous RV with exponential distribution and parameter $\lambda = 0.2$.

The exponential probability distribution is also a very important probability density function in biomedical engineering applications, arising in situations involving reliability theory and queuing problems. Reliability theory, which describes the time to failure for a system or component, grew primarily out of military applications and experiences with multicomponent systems. Queuing theory describes the waiting times between events.

The characteristic function can be found as

$$\phi_x(t) = \lambda \int_0^\infty e^{\alpha(jt-\lambda)} d\alpha = \frac{\lambda}{\lambda - jt}. \tag{5.16}$$

Figure 5.4 illustrates the PDF and the magnitude of the characteristic function for a continuous RV with exponential distribution and parameter $\lambda = 0.2$.

The mean and variance of a continuous exponentially distributed RV can be obtained using the moment generating property of the characteristic function. The results are

$$\eta_x = \frac{1}{\lambda}, \quad \sigma_x^2 = \frac{1}{\lambda^2}. \tag{5.17}$$

A continuous exponentially distributed RV, like its discrete counterpart, satisfies a memoryless property:

$$f_{x|x>\tau}(\alpha|x > \tau) = f_x(\alpha - \tau), \quad \tau \geq 0. \tag{5.18}$$

Example 5.2.1. *Suppose a system contains a component that has an exponential failure rate. Reliability engineers determined its reliability at 5000 hours to be 95%. Determine the number of hours reliable at 99%.*

Solution. First, the parameter λ is determined from

$$0.95 = P(x > 5000) = \int_{5000}^{\infty} \lambda e^{-\lambda \alpha} d\alpha = e^{-5000\lambda}.$$

Thus

$$\lambda = \frac{-\ln(0.95)}{5000} = 1.03 \times 10^{-5}.$$

Then, to determine the number of hours reliable at 99%, we solve for α from

$$P(x > \alpha) = e^{-\lambda \alpha} = 0.99$$

or

$$\alpha = \frac{-\ln(0.99)}{\lambda} = 980 \text{ hours.} \qquad \blacksquare$$

Drill Problem 5.2.1. *Suppose a system has an exponential failure rate in years to failure with $\lambda = 0.02$. Determine the number of years reliable at: (a) 90%, (b) 95%, (c) 99%.*

Answers: 0.5, 2.6, 5.3.

Drill Problem 5.2.2. *Random variable x, representing the length of time in hours to complete an examination in Introduction to Random Processes, has PDF*

$$f_x(\alpha) = \frac{4}{3} e^{-\frac{4}{3}\alpha} u(\alpha).$$

The examination results are given by

$$g(x) = \begin{cases} 75, & 0 < x < 4/3 \\ 75 + 39.44(x - 4/3), & x \geq 4/3 \\ 0, & \text{otherwise.} \end{cases}$$

Determine the average examination grade.

Answer: 80.

5.3 BERNOULLI TRIALS

A Bernoulli experiment consists of a number of repeated (independent) trials with only two possible events for each trial. The events for each trial can be thought of as any two events which partition the sample space, such as a head and a tail in a coin toss, a zero or one in a computer bit, or an even and odd number in a die toss. Let us call one of the events a success, the other a failure. The Bernoulli PMF describes the probability of k successes in n trials of a Bernoulli experiment. The first two chapters used this PMF repeatedly in problems dealing with games of chance and in situations where there were only two possible outcomes in any given trial. For biomedical engineers, the Bernoulli distribution is used in infectious disease problems and other applications. The Bernoulli distribution is also known as a Binomial distribution.

Definition 5.3.1. *A discrete RV x is **Bernoulli** distributed if the PMF for x is*

$$p_x(k) = \begin{cases} \binom{n}{k} p^k q^{n-k}, & k = 0, 1, \ldots, n \\ 0, & \text{otherwise,} \end{cases} \qquad (5.19)$$

where p = probability of success and $q = 1 - p$.

The characteristic function can be found using the binomial theorem:

$$\phi_x(t) = \sum_{k=0}^{n} \binom{n}{k} (pe^{jt})^k q^{n-k} = (q + pe^{jt})^n. \qquad (5.20)$$

Figure 5.5 illustrates the PMF and the characteristic function magnitude for a discrete RV with Bernoulli distribution, $p = 0.2$, and $n = 30$.

Using the moment generating property of characteristic functions, the mean and variance of a Bernoulli RV can be shown to be

$$\eta_x = np, \qquad \sigma_x^2 = npq. \qquad (5.21)$$

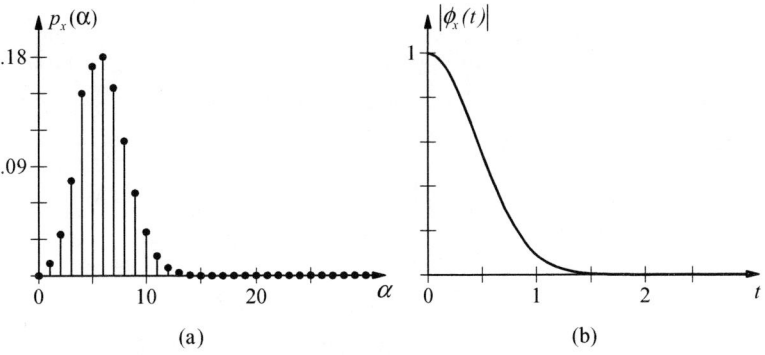

FIGURE 5.5: (a) PMF and (b) characteristic function magnitude for discrete RV with Bernoulli distribution, $p = 0.2$ and $n = 30$.

8 ADVANCED PROBABILITY THEORY FOR BIOMEDICAL ENGINEERS

Unlike the preceding distributions, a closed form expression for the Bernoulli CDF is not easily obtained. Tables A.1–A.3 in the Appendix list values of the Bernoulli CDF for $p = 0.05, 0.1, 0.15, \ldots, 0.5$ and $n = 5, 10, 15,$ and 20. Let $k \in \{0, 1, \ldots, n-1\}$ and define

$$G(n, k, p) = \sum_{\ell=0}^{k} \binom{n}{\ell} p^{\ell}(1-p)^{n-\ell}.$$

Making the change of variable $m = n - \ell$ yields

$$G(n, k, p) = \sum_{m=n-k}^{n} \binom{n}{n-m} p^{n-m}(1-p)^{m}.$$

Now, since

$$\binom{n}{n-m} = \frac{n!}{m!(n-m)!} = \binom{n}{m},$$

$$G(n, k, p) = \sum_{m=0}^{n} \binom{n}{m} p^{n-m}(1-p)^{m} - \sum_{m=0}^{n-k-1} \binom{n}{m} p^{n-m}(1-p)^{m}.$$

Using the Binomial Theorem,

$$G(n, k, p) = 1 - G(n, n-k-1, 1-p). \tag{5.22}$$

This result is easily applied to obtain values of the Bernoulli CDF for values of $p > 0.5$ from Tables A.1–A.3.

Example 5.3.1. *The probability that Fargo Polytechnic Institute wins a game is 0.7. In a 15 game season, what is the probability that they win: (a) at least 10 games, (b) from 9 to 12 games, (c) exactly 11 games? (d) With x denoting the number of games won, find η_x and σ_x^2.*

Solution. With x a Bernoulli random variable, we consult Table A.2, using (5.22) with $n = 15$, $k = 9$, and $p = 0.7$, we find

a) $P(x \geq 10) = 1 - F_x(9) = 1.0 - 0.2784 = 0.7216,$
b) $P(9 \leq x \leq 12) = F_x(12) - F_x(8) = 0.8732 - 0.1311 = 0.7421,$
c) $p_x(11) = F_x(11) - F_x(10) = 0.7031 - 0.4845 = 0.2186.$
d) $\eta_x = np = 10.5, \sigma_x^2 = np(1-p) = 3.15.$ ∎

STANDARD PROBABILITY DISTRIBUTIONS

We now consider the number of trials needed for k successes in a sequence of Bernoulli trials. Let

$$p(k, n) = P(k \text{ successes in } n \text{ trials}) \qquad (5.23)$$
$$= \begin{cases} \binom{n}{k} p^k q^{n-k}, & k = 0, 1, \ldots, n \\ 0, & \text{otherwise}, \end{cases}$$

where $p = p(1, 1)$ and $q = 1 - p$. Let RV n_r represent the number of trials to obtain exactly r successes ($r \geq 1$). Note that

$$P(\text{success in } \ell\text{th trial} \mid r - 1 \text{ successes in previous } \ell - 1 \text{ trials}) = p; \qquad (5.24)$$

hence, for $\ell = r, r + 1, \ldots$, we have

$$P(n_r = \ell) = p(r - 1, \ell - 1) p. \qquad (5.25)$$

Discrete RV n_r thus has PMF

$$p_{n_r}(\ell) = \begin{cases} \binom{\ell - 1}{r - 1} p^r q^{\ell - r}, & \ell = r, r + 1, \ldots \\ 0, & \text{otherwise}, \end{cases} \qquad (5.26)$$

where the parameter r is a positive integer. The PMF for the RV n_r is called the **negative binomial distribution**, also known as the Pólya and the Pascal distribution. Note that with $r = 1$ the negative binomial PMF is the geometric PMF.

The moment generating function for n_r can be expressed as

$$M_{n_r}(\lambda) = \sum_{\ell = r}^{\infty} \frac{(\ell - 1)(\ell - 2) \cdots (\ell - r + 1)}{(r - 1)!} p^r q^{\ell - r} e^{\lambda \ell}.$$

Letting $m = \ell - r$, we obtain

$$M_{n_r}(\lambda) = \frac{e^{\lambda r} p^r}{(r - 1)!} \sum_{m=0}^{\infty} (m + r - 1)(m + r - 2) \cdots (m + 1)(q e^\lambda)^m.$$

With

$$s(x) = \sum_{k=0}^{\infty} x^k = \frac{1}{1 - x}, \qquad |x| < 1,$$

we have

$$\begin{aligned}
s^{(\ell)}(x) &= \sum_{k=\ell}^{\infty} k(k-1)\cdots(k-\ell+1)x^{k-\ell} \\
&= \sum_{m=0}^{\infty} (m+\ell)(m+\ell-1)\cdots(m+1)x^m \\
&= \frac{\ell!}{(1-x)^{\ell+1}}.
\end{aligned}$$

Hence

$$M_{n_r}(\lambda) = \left(\frac{pe^\lambda}{1-qe^\lambda}\right)^r, \quad qe^\lambda < 1. \tag{5.27}$$

The mean and variance for n_r are found to be

$$\eta_{n_r} = \frac{r}{p}, \quad \text{and} \quad \sigma^2_{n_r} = \frac{rq}{p^2}. \tag{5.28}$$

We note that the characteristic function is simply

$$\phi_{n_r}(t) = M_{n_r}(jt) = \phi_x^r(t), \tag{5.29}$$

where RV x has a discrete geometric distribution. Figure 5.6 illustrates the PMF and the characteristic function magnitude for a discrete RV with negative binomial distribution, $r=3$, and $p=0.18127$.

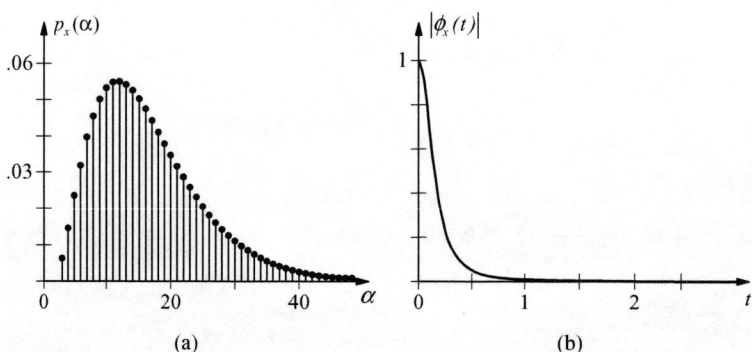

FIGURE 5.6: (a) PMF and (b) magnitude characteristic function for discrete RV with negative binomial distribution, $r=3$, and $p=0.18127$.

5.3.1 Poisson Approximation to Bernoulli

When n becomes large in the Bernoulli PMF in such a way that $np = \lambda = $ constant, the Bernoulli PMF approaches another important PMF known as the Poisson PMF. The Poisson PMF is treated in the following section.

Lemma 5.3.1. *We have*

$$p(k) = \lim_{n \to \infty, np=\lambda} \binom{n}{k} p^k q^{n-k} = \begin{cases} \dfrac{\lambda^k e^{-\lambda}}{k!}, & k = 0, 1, \ldots \\ 0, & \text{otherwise,} \end{cases} \qquad (5.30)$$

Proof. Substituting $p = \frac{\lambda}{n}$ and $q = 1 - \frac{\lambda}{n}$,

$$p(k) = \lim_{n \to \infty} \frac{1}{k!} \left(\frac{\lambda}{n}\right)^k \left(1 - \frac{\lambda}{n}\right)^{n-k} \prod_{i=0}^{k-1}(n-i).$$

Note that

$$\lim_{n \to \infty} n^{-k} \left(1 - \frac{\lambda}{n}\right)^{-k} \prod_{i=0}^{k-1}(n-i) = 1,$$

so that

$$p(k) = \lim_{n \to \infty} \frac{\lambda^k}{k!} \left(1 - \frac{\lambda}{n}\right)^n.$$

Now,

$$\lim_{n \to \infty} \ln\left(1 - \frac{\lambda}{n}\right)^n = \lim_{n \to \infty} \frac{\ln\left(1 - \frac{\lambda}{n}\right)}{\frac{1}{n}} = -\lambda$$

so that

$$\lim_{n \to \infty} \left(1 - \frac{\lambda}{n}\right)^n = e^{-\lambda},$$

from which the desired result follows. ∎

We note that the limiting value $p(k)$ may be used as an approximation for the Bernoulli PMF when p is small by substituting $\lambda = np$. While there are no prescribed rules regarding the values of n and p for this approximation, the larger the value of n and the smaller the value of p, the better the approximation. Satisfactory results are obtained with $np < 10$. The motivation for using this approximation is that when n is large, Tables A.1–A.3 are useless for finding values for the Bernoulli CDF.

12 ADVANCED PROBABILITY THEORY FOR BIOMEDICAL ENGINEERS

Example 5.3.2. *Suppose x is a Bernoulli random variable with $n = 5000$ and $p = 0.001$. Find $P(x \leq 5)$.*

Solution. Our solution involves approximating the Bernoulli PMF with the Poisson PMF since n is quite large (and the Bernoulli CDF table is useless), and p is very close to zero. Since $\lambda = np = 5$, we find from Table A.5 (the Poisson CDF table is covered in Section 4) that $P(x \leq 5) = 0.6160$. ∎

Incidentally, if p is close to one, we can still use this approximation by reversing our definition of success and failure in the Bernoulli experiment, which results in a value of p close to zero—see (5.22).

5.3.2 Gaussian Approximation to Bernoulli

Previously, the Poisson PMF was used to approximate a Bernoulli PMF under certain conditions, that is, when n is large, p is small and $np < 10$. This approximation is quite useful since the Bernoulli table lists only CDF values for n up to 20. The Gaussian PDF (see Section 5.5) is also used to approximate a Bernoulli PMF under certain conditions. The accuracy of this approximation is best when n is large, p is close to 1/2, and $npq > 3$. Notice that in some circumstances $np < 10$ and $npq > 3$. Then either the Poisson or the Gaussian approximation will yield good results.

Lemma 5.3.2. *Let*

$$y = \frac{x - np}{\sqrt{npq}}, \qquad (5.31)$$

where x is a Bernoulli RV. Then the characteristic function for y satisfies

$$\phi(t) = \lim_{n \to \infty} \phi_y(t) = e^{-t^2/2}. \qquad (5.32)$$

Proof. We have

$$\phi_y(t) = \exp\left(-j\frac{np}{\sqrt{npq}} t\right) \phi_x\left(\frac{t}{\sqrt{npq}}\right).$$

Substituting for $\phi_x(t)$,

$$\phi_y(t) = \exp\left(-j\sqrt{\frac{np}{q}} t\right) \left(q + p \exp\left(j\frac{t}{\sqrt{npq}}\right)\right)^n.$$

Simplifying,

$$\phi_y(t) = \left(q \exp\left(-jt\sqrt{\frac{p}{qn}}\right) + p \exp\left(jt\sqrt{\frac{q}{np}}\right)\right)^n.$$

Letting
$$\beta = \sqrt{\frac{q}{p}}, \quad \text{and} \quad \alpha = \sqrt{\frac{1}{n}},$$
we obtain
$$\lim_{n \to \infty} \ln \phi_y(t) = \lim_{\alpha \to 0} \frac{\ln(p\beta^2 e^{-jt\alpha/\beta} + p e^{jt\beta\alpha})}{\alpha^2}.$$

Applying L'Hôspital's Rule twice,
$$\lim_{\alpha \to 0} \ln \phi_y(t) = \lim_{\alpha \to 0} \frac{-jtp\beta e^{-jt\alpha/\beta} + jtp\beta e^{jt\beta\alpha}}{2\alpha} = \frac{-t^2 p - t^2 \beta^2 p}{2} = -\frac{t^2}{2}.$$

Consequently,
$$\lim_{n \to \infty} \phi_y(t) = \exp\left(\lim_{n \to \infty} \ln \phi_y(t)\right) = e^{-t^2/2}.$$

∎

The limiting $\phi(t)$ in the above lemma is the characteristic function for a Gaussian RV with zero mean and unit variance. Hence, for large n and $a < b$
$$P(a < x < b) = P(a' < y < b') \approx F(b') - F(a'), \tag{5.33}$$
where
$$F(\gamma) = \frac{1}{\sqrt{2\pi}} \int_{-\infty}^{\gamma} e^{-\alpha^2/2} d\alpha = 1 - Q(\gamma) \tag{5.34}$$
is the standard Gaussian CDF,
$$a' = \frac{a - np}{\sqrt{npq}}, \qquad b' = \frac{b - np}{\sqrt{npq}}, \tag{5.35}$$
and $Q(\cdot)$ is Marcum's Q function which is tabulated in Tables A.8 and A.9 of the Appendix. Evaluation of the above integral as well as the Gaussian PDF are treated in Section 5.5.

Example 5.3.3. *Suppose x is a Bernoulli random variable with $n = 5000$ and $p = 0.4$. Find $P(x \leq 2048)$.*

Solution. The solution involves approximating the Bernoulli CDF with the Gaussian CDF since $npq = 1200 > 3$. With $np = 2000$, $npq = 1200$ and $b' = (2048 - 2000)/34.641 = 1.39$, we find from Table A.8 that
$$P(x \leq 2048) \approx F(1.39) = 1 - Q(1.39) = 0.91774.$$
∎

14 ADVANCED PROBABILITY THEORY FOR BIOMEDICAL ENGINEERS

When approximating the Bernoulli CDF with the Gaussian CDF, a continuous distribution is used to calculate probabilities for a discrete RV. It is important to note that while the approximation is excellent in terms of the CDFs—the PDF of any discrete RV is never approximated with a continuous PDF. Operationally, to compute the probability that a Bernoulli RV takes an integer value using the Gaussian approximation we must round off to the nearest integer.

Example 5.3.4. *Suppose x is a Bernoulli random variable with $n = 20$ and $p = 0.5$. Find $P(x = 8)$.*

Solution. Since $npq = 5 > 3$, the Gaussian approximation is used to evaluate the Bernoulli PMF, $p_x(8)$. With $np = 10$, $npq = 5$, $a' = (7.5 - 10)/\sqrt{5} = -1.12$, and $b' = (8.5 - 10)/\sqrt{5} = -0.67$, we have

$$p_x(8) = P(7.5 < x < 8.5) \approx F(-0.67) - F(-1.12) = 0.25143 - 0.13136;$$

hence, $p_x(8) \approx 0.12007$. From the Bernoulli table, $p_x(8) = 0.1201$, which is very close to the above approximation. ∎

Drill Problem 5.3.1. *A survey of residents in Fargo, North Dakota revealed that 30% preferred a white automobile over all other colors. Determine the probability that: (a) exactly five of the next 20 cars purchased will be white, (b) at least five of the next twenty cars purchased will be white, (c) from two to five of the next twenty cars purchased will be white.*

Answers: 0.1789, 0.4088, 0.7625.

Drill Problem 5.3.2. *Prof. Rensselaer is an avid albeit inaccurate marksman. The probability she will hit the target is only 0.3. Determine: (a) the expected number of hits scored in 15 shots, (b) the standard deviation for 15 shots, (c) the number of times she must fire so that the probability of hitting the target at least once is greater than 1/2.*

Answers: 2, 4.5, 1.7748.

5.4 POISSON DISTRIBUTION

A Poisson PMF describes the number of successes occurring on a continuous line, typically a time interval, or within a given region. For example, a Poisson random variable might represent the number of telephone calls per hour, or the number of errors per page in this textbook.

In the previous section, we found that the limit (as $n \to \infty$ and constant mean np) of a Bernoulli PMF is a Poisson PMF. In this section, we derive the Poisson probability distribution from two fundamental assumptions about the phenomenon based on physical characteristics.

STANDARD PROBABILITY DISTRIBUTIONS   15

The following development makes use of the order notation $o(h)$ to denote **any** function $g(h)$ which satisfies

$$\lim_{h \to 0} \frac{g(h)}{h} = 0. \tag{5.36}$$

For example, $g(h) = 15h^2 + 7h^3 = o(h)$.

We use the notation

$$p(k, \tau) = P(k \text{ successes in interval } [0, \tau]). \tag{5.37}$$

The Poisson probability distribution is characterized by the following two properties:

(1) The number of successes occurring in a time interval or region is independent of the number of successes occurring in any other non-overlapping time interval or region. Thus, with

$$A = \{k \text{ successes in interval } I_1\}, \tag{5.38}$$

and

$$B = \{\ell \text{ successes in interval } I_2\}, \tag{5.39}$$

we have

$$P(A \cap B) = P(A)P(B), \quad \text{if } I_1 \cap I_2 = \Phi. \tag{5.40}$$

As we will see, the number of successes depends only on the length of the time interval and not the location of the interval on the time axis.

(2) The probability of a single success during a very small time interval is proportional to the length of the interval. The longer the interval, the greater the probability of success. The probability of more than one success occurring during an interval vanishes as the length of the interval approaches zero. Hence

$$p(1, h) = \lambda h + o(h), \tag{5.41}$$

and

$$p(0, h) = 1 - \lambda h + o(h). \tag{5.42}$$

This second property indicates that for a series of very small intervals, the Poisson process is composed of a series of Bernoulli trials, each with a probability of success $p = \lambda h + o(h)$.

Since $[0, \tau + h] = [0, \tau] \cup (\tau, \tau + h]$ and $[0, \tau] \cap (\tau, \tau + h] = \Phi$, we have

$$p(0, \tau + h) = p(0, \tau)p(0, h) = p(0, \tau)(1 - \lambda h + o(h)).$$

16   ADVANCED PROBABILITY THEORY FOR BIOMEDICAL ENGINEERS

Noting that

$$\frac{p(0,\tau+h)-p(0,\tau)}{h} = \frac{-\lambda h p(0,\tau) + o(h)}{h}$$

and taking the limit as $h \to 0$,

$$\frac{dp(0,\tau)}{d\tau} = -\lambda p(0,\tau), \quad p(0,0) = 1. \quad (5.43)$$

This differential equation has solution

$$p(0,\tau) = e^{-\lambda\tau} u(\tau). \quad (5.44)$$

Applying the above properties, it is readily seen that

$$p(k,\tau+h) = p(k-1,\tau)p(1,h) + p(k,\tau)p(0,h) + o(h),$$

or

$$p(k,\tau+h) = p(k-1,\tau)\lambda h + p(k,\tau)(1-\lambda h) + o(h),$$

so that

$$\frac{p(k,\tau+h) - p(k,\tau)}{h} + \lambda p(k,\tau) = \lambda p(k-1,\tau) + \frac{o(h)}{h}.$$

Taking the limit as $h \to 0$

$$\frac{dp(k,\tau)}{d\tau} + \lambda p(k,\tau) = \lambda p(k-1,\tau), \quad k = 1, 2, \ldots, \quad (5.45)$$

with $p(k,0) = 0$. It can be shown ([7, 8]) that

$$p(k,\tau) = \lambda e^{-\lambda\tau} \int_0^\tau e^{\lambda t} p(k-1,t) dt \quad (5.46)$$

and hence that

$$p(k,\tau) = \frac{(\lambda\tau)^k e^{-\lambda\tau}}{k!} u(\tau), \quad k = 0, 1, \ldots. \quad (5.47)$$

The RV x = number of successes thus has a Poisson distribution with parameter $\lambda\tau$ and PMF $p_x(k) = p(k,\tau)$. The rate of the Poisson process is λ and the interval length is τ.

For ease in subsequent development, we replace the parameter $\lambda\tau$ with λ. The characteristic function for a Poisson RV x with parameter λ is found as (with parameter λ, $p_x(k) = p(k,1)$)

$$\phi_x(t) = e^{-\lambda} \sum_{k=0}^\infty \frac{(\lambda e^{jt})^k}{k!} = e^{-\lambda} \exp(\lambda e^{jt}) = \exp(\lambda(e^{jt}-1)). \quad (5.48)$$

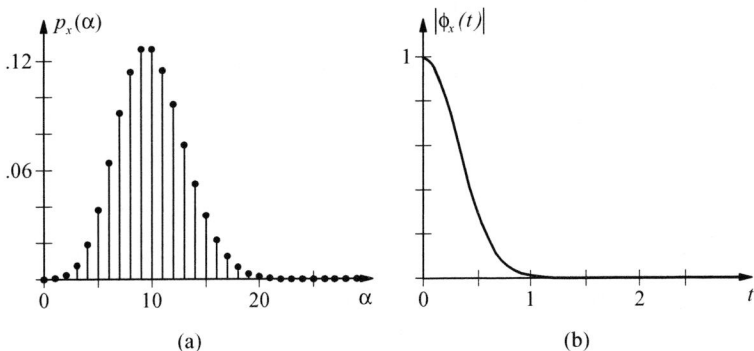

FIGURE 5.7: (a) PMF and (b) magnitude characteristic function for Poisson distributed RV with parameter $\lambda = 10$.

Figure 5.7 illustrates the PMF and characteristic function magnitude for a discrete RV with Poisson distribution and parameter $\lambda = 10$.

It is of interest to note that if x_1 and x_2 are independent Poisson RVs with parameters λ_1 and λ_2, respectively, then

$$\phi_{x_1+x_2}(t) = \exp((\lambda_1 + \lambda_2)(e^{jt} - 1)); \qquad (5.49)$$

i.e., $x_1 + x_2$ is also a Poisson with parameter $\lambda_1 + \lambda_2$.

The moments of a Poisson RV are tedious to compute using techniques we have seen so far. Consider the function

$$\psi_x(\gamma) = E(\gamma^x) \qquad (5.50)$$

and note that

$$\psi_x^{(k)}(\gamma) = E\left(\gamma^{x-k} \prod_{i=0}^{k-1}(x-i)\right),$$

so that

$$E\left(\prod_{i=0}^{k-1}(x-i)\right) = \psi_x^{(k)}(1). \qquad (5.51)$$

If x is Poisson distributed with parameter λ, then

$$\psi_x(\gamma) = e^{\lambda(\gamma-1)}, \qquad (5.52)$$

so that

$$\psi_x^{(k)}(\gamma) = \lambda^k e^{\lambda(\gamma-1)};$$

hence,

$$E\left(\prod_{i=0}^{k-1}(x-i)\right) = \lambda^k. \qquad (5.53)$$

In particular, $E(x) = \lambda$, $E(x(x-1)) = \lambda^2 = E(x^2) - \lambda$, so that $\sigma_x^2 = \lambda^2 + \lambda - \lambda^2 = \lambda$.

While it is quite easy to calculate the value of the Poisson PMF for a particular number of successes, hand computation of the CDF is quite tedious. Therefore, the Poisson CDF is tabulated in Tables A.4-A.7 of the Appendix for selected values of λ ranging from 0.1 to 18. From the Poisson CDF table, we note that the value of the Poisson PMF increases as the number of successes k increases from zero to the mean, and then decreases in value as k increases from the mean. Additionally, note that the table is written with a finite number of entries for each value of λ because the PMF values are written with six decimal place accuracy, even though an infinite number of Poisson successes are theoretically possible.

Example 5.4.1. *On the average, Professor Rensselaer grades 10 problems per day. What is the probability that on a given day (a) 8 problems are graded, (b) 8–10 problems are graded, and (c) at least 15 problems are graded?*

Solution. With x a Poisson random variable, we consult the Poisson CDF table with $\lambda = 10$, and find

a) $p_x(8) = F_x(8) - F_x(7) = 0.3328 - 0.2202 = 0.1126,$
b) $P(8 \leq x \leq 10) = F_x(10) - F_x(7) = 0.5830 - 0.2202 = 0.3628,$
c) $P(x \geq 15) = 1 - F_x(14) = 1 - 0.9165 = 0.0835.$ ∎

5.4.1 Interarrival Times

In many instances, the length of time between successes, known as an interarrival time, of a Poisson random variable is more important than the actual number of successes. For example, in evaluating the reliability of a medical device, the time to failure is far more significant to the biomedical engineer than the fact that the device failed. Indeed, the subject of reliability theory is so important that entire textbooks are devoted to the topic. Here, however, we will briefly examine the subject of interarrival times from the basis of the Poisson PMF.

Let RV t_r denote the length of the time interval from zero to the rth success. Then

$$p(\tau - h < t_r \leq \tau) = p(r-1, \tau-h)p(1, h)$$
$$= p(r-1, \tau-h)\lambda h + o(h)$$

so that
$$\frac{F_{t_r}(\tau) - F_{t_r}(\tau - h)}{h} = \lambda p(r-1, \tau - h) + \frac{o(h)}{h}.$$

Taking the limit as $h \to 0$ we find that the PDF for the rth order interarrival time, that is, the time interval from any starting point to the rth success after it, is

$$f_{t_r}(\tau) = \frac{\lambda^r \tau^{r-1} e^{-\lambda \tau}}{(r-1)!} u(\tau), \quad r = 1, 2, \ldots. \tag{5.54}$$

This PDF is known as the Erlang PDF. Clearly, with $r = 1$, we have the exponential PDF:

$$f_t(\tau) = \lambda e^{-\lambda \tau} u(\tau). \tag{5.55}$$

The RV t is called the first-order interarrival time.

The Erlang PDF is a special case of the gamma PDF:

$$f_x(\alpha) = \frac{\lambda^r \alpha^{r-1} e^{-\lambda \alpha}}{\Gamma(r)} u(\alpha), \tag{5.56}$$

for any real $r > 0$, $\lambda > 0$, where Γ is the gamma function

$$\Gamma(r) = \int_0^\infty \alpha^{r-1} e^{-\alpha} d\alpha. \tag{5.57}$$

Straightforward integration reveals that $\Gamma(1) = 1$ and $\Gamma(r+1) = r\Gamma(r)$ so that if r is a positive integer then $\Gamma(r) = (r-1)!$—for this reason the gamma function is often called the factorial function. Using the above definition for $\Gamma(r)$, it is easily shown that the moment generating function for a gamma-distributed RV is

$$M_x(\eta) = \left(\frac{\lambda}{\lambda - \eta}\right)^r, \quad \text{for} \quad \eta < \lambda. \tag{5.58}$$

The characteristic function is thus

$$\phi_x(t) = \left(\frac{\lambda}{\lambda - jt}\right)^r. \tag{5.59}$$

It follows that the mean and variance are

$$\eta_x = \frac{r}{\lambda}, \quad \text{and} \quad \sigma_x^2 = \frac{r}{\lambda^2}. \tag{5.60}$$

Figure 5.8 illustrates the PDF and magnitude of the characteristic function for a RV with gamma distribution with $r = 3$ and $\lambda = 0.2$.

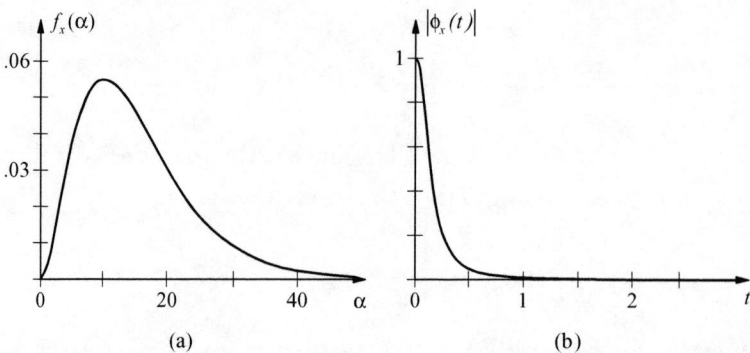

FIGURE 5.8: (a) PDF and (b) magnitude characteristic function for gamma distributed RV with $r = 3$ and parameter $\lambda = 0.2$.

Drill Problem 5.4.1. *On the average, Professor S. Rensselaer makes five blunders per lecture. Determine the probability that she makes (a) less than six blunders in the next lecture: (b) exactly five blunders in the next lecture: (c) from three to seven blunders in the next lecture: (d) zero blunders in the next lecture.*

Answers: 0.6160, 0.0067, 0.7419, 0.1755.

Drill Problem 5.4.2. *A process yields 0.001% defective items. If one million items are produced, determine the probability that the number of defective items exceeds twelve.*

Answer: 0.2084.

Drill Problem 5.4.3. *Professor S. Rensselaer designs her examinations so that the probability of at least one extremely difficult problem is 0.632. Determine the average number of extremely difficult problems on a Rensselaer examination.*

Answer: 1.

5.5 UNIVARIATE GAUSSIAN DISTRIBUTION

The Gaussian PDF is the most important probability distribution in the field of biomedical engineering. Plentiful applications arise in industry, research, and nature, ranging from instrumentation errors to scores on examinations. The PDF is named in honor of Gauss (1777–1855), who derived the equation based on an error study involving repeated measurements of the same quantity. However, De Moivre is first credited with describing the PDF in 1733. Applications also abound in other areas outside of biomedical engineering since the distribution fits the observed data in many processes. Incidentally, statisticians refer to the Gaussian PDF as the normal PDF.

Definition 5.5.1. *A continuous RV z is a **standardized Gaussian** RV if the PDF is*

$$f_z(\alpha) = \frac{1}{\sqrt{2\pi}} e^{-\frac{1}{2}\alpha^2}. \qquad (5.61)$$

The moment generating function for a standardized Gaussian RV can be found as follows:

$$M_z(\lambda) = \frac{1}{\sqrt{2\pi}} \int_{-\infty}^{\infty} e^{\lambda\alpha - \frac{1}{2}\alpha^2} d\alpha$$

$$= \frac{1}{\sqrt{2\pi}} \int_{-\infty}^{\infty} e^{-\frac{1}{2}((\alpha-\lambda)^2 - \lambda^2)} d\alpha.$$

Making the change of variable $\beta = \alpha - \lambda$ we find

$$M_z(\lambda) = e^{\frac{1}{2}\lambda^2} \int_{-\infty}^{\infty} f_z(\beta) d\beta = e^{\frac{1}{2}\lambda^2}, \qquad (5.62)$$

for all real λ. We have made use of the fact that the function f_z is a bona fide PDF, as treated in Problem 42. Using the Taylor series expansion for an exponential,

$$e^{\frac{1}{2}\lambda^2} = \sum_{k=0}^{\infty} \frac{\lambda^{2k}}{2^k k!} = \sum_{n=0}^{\infty} \frac{M_x^{(n)}(0)\lambda^n}{n!},$$

so that all moments of z exist and

$$E(z^{2k}) = \frac{(2k)!}{2^k k!}, \qquad k = 0, 1, 2, \ldots, \qquad (5.63)$$

and

$$E(z^{2k+1}) = 0, \qquad k = 0, 1, 2, \ldots. \qquad (5.64)$$

Consequently, a standardized Gaussian RV has zero mean and unit variance. Extending the range of definition of $M_z(\lambda)$ to include the finite complex plane, we find that the characteristic function is

$$\phi_z(t) = M_z(jt) = e^{-\frac{1}{2}t^2}. \qquad (5.65)$$

Letting the RV $x = \sigma z + \eta$ we find that $E(x) = \eta$ and $\sigma_x^2 = \sigma^2$. For $\sigma > 0$

$$F_x(\alpha) = P(\sigma z + \eta \leq \alpha) = F_z((\alpha - \eta)/\sigma),$$

so that x has the general **Gaussian** PDF

$$f_x(\alpha) = \frac{1}{\sqrt{2\pi\sigma^2}} \exp\left(-\frac{1}{2\sigma^2}(\alpha - \eta)^2\right). \qquad (5.66)$$

Similarly, with $\sigma > 0$ and $x = -\sigma z + \eta$ we find

$$F_x(\alpha) = P(-\sigma z + \eta \leq \alpha) = 1 - F_z((\eta - \alpha)/\sigma),$$

so that f_x is as above. We will have occasion to use the shorthand notation $x \sim G(\eta, \sigma^2)$ to denote that the RV has a Gaussian PDF with mean η and variance σ^2. Note that if $x \sim G(\eta, \sigma^2)$ then ($x = \sigma z + \eta$)

$$\phi_x(t) = e^{j\eta t} e^{-\frac{1}{2}\sigma^2 t^2}. \qquad (5.67)$$

The Gaussian PDF, illustrated with $\eta = 75$ and $\sigma^2 = 25$, as well as with $\eta = 75$ and $\sigma^2 = 9$ in Figure 5.9, is a bell-shaped curve completely determined by its mean and variance. As can be seen, the Gaussian PDF is symmetrical about the vertical axis through the expected value. If, in fact, $\eta = 25$, identically shaped curves could be drawn, centered now at 25 instead of 75. Additionally, the maximum value of the Gaussian PDF, $(2\pi\sigma^2)^{-1/2}$, occurs at $\alpha = \eta$. The PDF approaches zero asymptotically as α approaches $\pm\infty$. Naturally, the larger the value of the variance, the more spread in the distribution and the smaller the maximum value of the PDF. For any combination of the mean and variance, the Gaussian PDF curve must be symmetrical as previously described, and the area under the curve must equal one.

Unfortunately, a closed form expression does not exist for the Gaussian CDF, which necessitates numerical integration. Rather than attempting to tabulate the general Gaussian CDF, a normalization is performed to obtain a standardized Gaussian RV (with zero mean

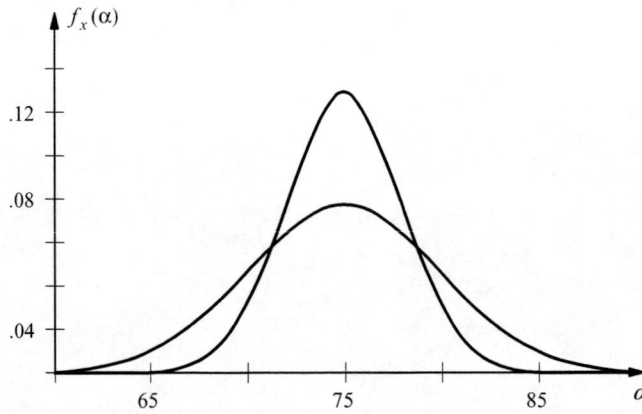

FIGURE 5.9: Gaussian probability density function for $\eta = 75$ and $\sigma^2 = 9, 25$.

STANDARD PROBABILITY DISTRIBUTIONS

and unit variance). If $x \sim G(\eta, \sigma^2)$, the RV $z = (x - \eta)/\sigma$ is a standardized Gaussian RV: $z \sim G(0, 1)$. This transformation is always applied when using standard tables for computing probabilities for Gaussian RVs. The probability $P(\alpha_1 < x \leq \alpha_2)$ can be obtained as

$$P(\alpha_1 < x \leq \alpha_2) = F_x(\alpha_2) - F_x(\alpha_1), \qquad (5.68)$$

using the fact that

$$F_x(\alpha) = F_z((\alpha - \eta)/\sigma). \qquad (5.69)$$

Note that

$$F_z(\alpha) = \frac{1}{\sqrt{2\pi}} \int_{-\infty}^{\alpha} e^{-\frac{1}{2}\tau^2} d\tau = 1 - Q(\alpha), \qquad (5.70)$$

where $Q(\cdot)$ is Marcum's Q function:

$$Q(\alpha) = \frac{1}{\sqrt{2\pi}} \int_{\alpha}^{\infty} e^{-\frac{1}{2}\tau^2} d\tau. \qquad (5.71)$$

Marcum's Q function is tabulated in Tables A.8 and A.9 for $0 \leq \alpha < 4$ using the approximation presented in Section 5.5.1. It is easy to show that

$$Q(-\alpha) = 1 - Q(\alpha) = F_z(\alpha). \qquad (5.72)$$

The error and complementary error functions, defined by

$$\mathrm{erf}(\alpha) = \frac{2}{\pi} \int_0^{\alpha} e^{-t^2} dt \qquad (5.73)$$

and

$$\mathrm{erfc}(\alpha) = \frac{2}{\pi} \int_{\alpha}^{\infty} e^{-t^2} dt = 1 - \mathrm{erf}(\alpha) \qquad (5.74)$$

are also often used to evaluate the standard normal integral. A simple change of variable reveals that

$$\mathrm{erfc}(\alpha) = 2Q(\alpha/\sqrt{2}). \qquad (5.75)$$

Example 5.5.1. *Compute $F_z(-1.74)$, where $z \sim G(0, 1)$.*

Solution. To compute $F_z(-1.74)$, we find

$$F_z(-1.74) = 1 - Q(-1.74) = Q(1.74) = 0.04093,$$

using (5.72) and Table A.8. ∎

While the value a Gaussian random variable takes on is any real number between negative infinity and positive infinity, the realistic range of values is much smaller. From Table A.9, we note that 99.73% of the area under the curve is contained between -3.0 and 3.0. From the transformation $z = (x - \eta)/\sigma$, the range of values random variable x takes on is then approximately $\eta \pm 3\sigma$. This notion does not imply that random variable x cannot take on a value outside this interval, but the probability of it occurring is really very small ($2Q(3) = 0.0027$).

Example 5.5.2. *Suppose x is a Gaussian random variable with $\eta = 35$ and $\sigma = 10$. Sketch the PDF and then find $P(37 \leq x \leq 51)$. Indicate this probability on the sketch.*

Solution. The PDF is essentially zero outside the interval $[\eta - 3\sigma, \eta + 3\sigma] = [5, 65]$. The sketch of this PDF is shown in Figure 5.10 along with the indicated probability. With

$$z = \frac{x - 35}{10}$$

we have

$$P(37 \leq x \leq 51) = P(0.2 \leq z \leq 1.6) = F_z(1.6) - F_z(0.2).$$

Hence $P(37 \leq x \leq 51) = Q(0.2) - Q(1.6) = 0.36594$ from Table A.9. ∎

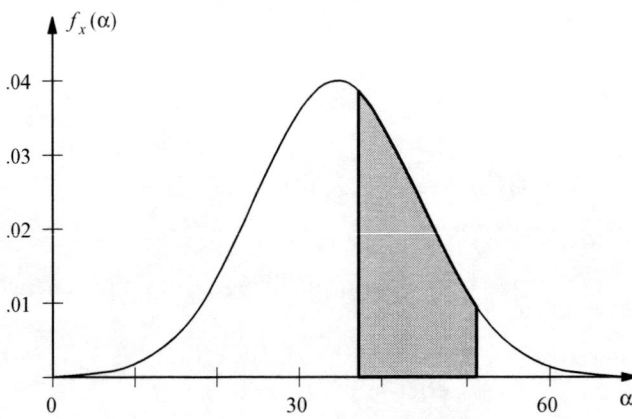

FIGURE 5.10: PDF for Example 5.5.2.

Example 5.5.3. *A machine makes capacitors with a mean value of 25 µF and a standard deviation of 6 µF. Assuming that capacitance follows a Gaussian distribution, find the probability that the value of capacitance exceeds 31 µF if capacitance is measured to the nearest µF.*

Solution. Let the RV x denote the value of a capacitor. Since we are measuring to the nearest µF, the probability that the measured value exceeds 31 µF is

$$P(31.5 \leq x) = P(1.083 \leq z) = Q(1.083) = 0.13941,$$

where $z = (x - 25)/6 \sim G(0, 1)$. This result is determined by linear interpolation of the CDF between equal 1.08 and 1.09. ∎

5.5.1 Marcum's Q Function

Marcum's Q function, defined by

$$Q(\gamma) = \frac{1}{\sqrt{2\pi}} \int_{\gamma}^{\infty} e^{-\frac{1}{2}\alpha^2} d\alpha \qquad (5.76)$$

has been extensively studied. If the RV $z \sim G(0, 1)$ then

$$Q(\gamma) = 1 - F_z(\gamma); \qquad (5.77)$$

i.e., $Q(\gamma)$ is the complement of the standard Gaussian CDF. Note that $Q(0) = 0.5$, $Q(\infty) = 0$, and that $F_z(-\gamma) = Q(\gamma)$. A very accurate approximation to $Q(\gamma)$ is presented in [1, p. 932]:

$$Q(\gamma) \approx e^{-\frac{1}{2}\gamma^2} h(t), \qquad \gamma > 0, \qquad (5.78)$$

where

$$t = \frac{1}{1 + 0.2316419\gamma}, \qquad (5.79)$$

and

$$h(t) = \frac{1}{\sqrt{2\pi}} t(a_1 + t(a_2 + t(a_3 + t(a_4 + a_5 t)))). \qquad (5.80)$$

The constants are

i	a_i
1	0.31938153
2	−0.356563782
3	1.781477937
4	−1.821255978
5	1.330274429

The error in using this approximation is less than 7.5×10^{-8}.

A very useful bound for $Q(\alpha)$ is [1, p. 298]

$$\sqrt{\frac{2}{\pi}} \frac{e^{-\frac{1}{2}\alpha^2}}{\alpha + \sqrt{\alpha^2 + 4}} < Q(\alpha) \leq \sqrt{\frac{2}{\pi}} \frac{e^{-\frac{1}{2}\alpha^2}}{\alpha + \sqrt{\alpha^2 + 0.5\pi}}. \qquad (5.81)$$

The ratio of the upper bound to the lower bound is 0.946 when $\alpha = 3$ and 0.967 when $\alpha = 4$. The bound improves as α increases.

Sometimes, it is desired to find the value of γ for which $Q(\gamma) = q$. Helstrom [14] offers an iterative procedure which begins with an initial guess $\gamma_0 > 0$. Then compute

$$t_i = \frac{1}{1 + 0.2316419\gamma_i} \qquad (5.82)$$

and

$$\gamma_{i+1} = \left(2\ln\left(\frac{h(t_i)}{q}\right)\right)^{1/2}, \qquad i = 0, 1, \ldots. \qquad (5.83)$$

The procedure is terminated when $\gamma_{i+1} \approx \gamma_i$ to the desired degree of accuracy.

Drill Problem 5.5.1. *Students attend Fargo Polytechnic Institute for an average of four years with a standard deviation of one-half year. Let the random variable x denote the length of attendance and assume that x is Gaussian. Determine: (a) $P(1 < x < 3)$, (b) $P(x > 4)$, (c) $P(x = 4)$, (d) $F_x(4.721)$.*

Answers: 0.5, 0, 0.02275, 0.92535.

Drill Problem 5.5.2. *The quality point averages of 2500 freshmen at Fargo Polytechnic Institute follow a Gaussian distribution with a mean of 2.5 and a standard deviation of 0.7. Suppose grade point averages are computed to the nearest tenth. Determine the number of freshmen you would expect to score: (a) from 2.6 to 3.0, (b) less than 2.5, (c) between 3.0 and 3.5, (d) greater than 3.5.*

Answers: 167, 322, 639, 1179.

Drill Problem 5.5.3. *Professor Rensselaer loves the game of golf. She has determined that the distance the ball travels on her first shot follows a Gaussian distribution with a mean of 150 and a standard deviation of 17. Determine the value of d so that the range, $150 \pm d$, covers 95% of the shots.*

Answer: 33.32.

5.6 BIVARIATE GAUSSIAN RANDOM VARIABLES

The previous section introduced the univariate Gaussian PDF along with some general characteristics. Now, we discuss the joint Gaussian PDF and its characteristics by drawing on our univariate Gaussian PDF experiences, and significantly expanding the scope of applications.

Numerous applications of this joint PDF are found throughout the field of biomedical engineering and, like the univariate case, the joint Gaussian PDF is considered the most important joint distribution for biomedical engineers.

Definition 5.6.1. *The bivariate RV* $\mathbf{z} = (x, y)$ *is a* **bivariate Gaussian** *RV if every linear combination of x and y has a univariate Gaussian distribution. In this case we also say that the RVs x and y are jointly distributed Gaussian RVs.*

Let the RV $w = ax + by$, and let x and y be jointly distributed Gaussian RVs. Then w is a univariate Gaussian RV for all real constants a and b. In particular, $x \sim G(\eta_x, \sigma_x^2)$ and $y \sim G(\eta_y, \sigma_y^2)$; i.e., the marginal PDFs for a joint Gaussian PDF are univariate Gaussian. The above definition of a bivariate Gaussian RV is sufficient for determining the bivariate PDF, which we now proceed to do.

The following development is significantly simplified by considering the standardized versions of x and y. Also, we assume that $|\rho_{x,y}| < 1$, $\sigma_x \neq 0$, and $\sigma_y \neq 0$. Let

$$z_1 = \frac{x - \eta_x}{\sigma_x} \quad \text{and} \quad z_2 = \frac{y - \eta_y}{\sigma_y}, \tag{5.84}$$

so that $z_1 \sim G(0, 1)$ and $z_2 \sim G(0, 1)$. Below, we first find the joint characteristic function for the standardized RVs z_1 and z_2, then the conditional PDF $f_{z_2|z_1}$ and the joint PDF f_{z_1,z_2}. Next, the results for z_1 and z_2 are applied to obtain corresponding quantities $\phi_{x,y}$, $f_{y|x}$ and $f_{x,y}$. Finally, the special cases $\rho_{x,y} = \pm 1$, $\sigma_x = 0$, and $\sigma_y = 0$ are discussed.

Since z_1 and z_2 are jointly Gaussian, the RV $t_1 z_1 + t_2 z_2$ is univariate Gaussian:

$$t_1 z_1 + t_2 z_2 \sim G\big(0, t_1^2 + 2 t_1 t_2 \rho + t_2^2\big).$$

Completing the square,

$$t_1^2 + 2 t_1 t_2 \rho + t_2^2 = (t_1 + \rho t_2)^2 + (1 - \rho^2) t_2^2,$$

so that

$$\phi_{z_1, z_2}(t_1, t_2) = E(e^{j t_1 z_1 + j t_2 z_2}) = e^{-\frac{1}{2}(1 - \rho^2) t_2^2} e^{-\frac{1}{2}(t_1 + \rho t_2)^2}. \tag{5.85}$$

From (6) we have

$$f_{z_1, z_2}(\alpha, \beta) = \frac{1}{2\pi} \int_{-\infty}^{\infty} I(\alpha, t_2) e^{-j \beta t_2} dt_2, \tag{5.86}$$

where

$$I(\alpha, t_2) = \frac{1}{2\pi} \int_{-\infty}^{\infty} \phi_{z_1,z_2}(t_1, t_2) e^{-j\alpha t_1} dt_1.$$

Substituting (5.85) and letting $\tau = t_1 + t_2\rho$, we obtain

$$I(\alpha, t_2) = e^{-\frac{1}{2}(1-\rho^2)t_2^2} \frac{1}{2\pi} \int_{-\infty}^{\infty} e^{-\frac{1}{2}\tau^2} e^{-j\alpha(\tau-\rho t_2)} d\tau,$$

or

$$I(\alpha, t_2) = \phi(t_2) f_{z_1}(\alpha),$$

where

$$\phi(t_2) = e^{j\alpha\rho t_2} e^{-\frac{1}{2}(1-\rho^2)t_2^2}.$$

Substituting into (5.86) we find

$$f_{z_1,z_2}(\alpha, \beta) = f_{z_1}(\alpha) \frac{1}{2\pi} \int_{-\infty}^{\infty} \phi(t_2) e^{-j\beta t_2} dt_2$$

and recognize that ϕ is the characteristic function for a Gaussian RV with mean $\alpha\rho$ and variance $1 - \rho^2$. Thus

$$\frac{f_{z_1,z_2}(\alpha, \beta)}{f_{z_1}(\alpha)} = f_{z_2|z_1}(\beta|\alpha) = \frac{1}{\sqrt{2\pi(1-\rho^2)}} \exp\left(-\frac{(\beta - \rho\alpha)^2}{2(1-\rho^2)}\right), \quad (5.87)$$

so that

$$E(z_2 \mid z_1) = \rho z_1 \quad (5.88)$$

and

$$\sigma^2_{z_2|z_1} = 1 - \rho^2. \quad (5.89)$$

After some algebra, we find

$$f_{z_1,z_2}(\alpha, \beta) = \frac{1}{2\pi(1-\rho^2)^{1/2}} \exp\left(-\frac{\alpha^2 - 2\rho\alpha\beta + \beta^2}{2(1-\rho^2)}\right). \quad (5.90)$$

We now turn our attention to using the above results for z_1 and z_2 to obtain similar results for x and y. From (5.84) we find that

$$x = \sigma_x z_1 + \eta_x \quad \text{and} \quad y = \sigma_y z_2 + \eta_y,$$

so that the joint characteristic function for x and y is

$$\phi_{x,y}(t_1, t_2) = E(e^{jt_1 x + jt_2 y}) = E(e^{jt_1 \sigma_x z_1 + jt_2 \sigma_y z_2}) e^{jt_1 \eta_x + jt_2 \eta_y}.$$

Consequently, the joint characteristic function for x and y can be found from the joint characteristic function of z_1 and z_2 as

$$\phi_{x,y}(t_1, t_2) = \phi_{z_1, z_2}(\sigma_x t_1, \sigma_y t_2) e^{j\eta_x t_1} e^{j\eta_y t_2}. \tag{5.91}$$

Using (4.66), the joint characteristic function $\phi_{x,y}$ can be transformed to obtain the joint PDF $f_{x,y}(\alpha, \beta)$ as

$$f_{x,y}(\alpha, \beta) = \frac{1}{(2\pi)^2} \int_{-\infty}^{\infty} \int_{-\infty}^{\infty} \phi_{z_1, z_2}(\sigma_x t_1, \sigma_y t_2) e^{-j(\alpha - \eta_x) t_1} e^{-j(\beta - \eta_y) t_2} dt_1 dt_2. \tag{5.92}$$

Making the change of variables $\tau_1 = \sigma_x t_1$, $\tau_2 = \sigma_y t_2$, we obtain

$$f_{x,y}(\alpha, \beta) = \frac{1}{\sigma_x \sigma_y} f_{z_1, z_2}\left(\frac{\alpha - \eta_x}{\sigma_x}, \frac{\beta - \eta_y}{\sigma_y}\right). \tag{5.93}$$

Since

$$f_{x,y}(\alpha, \beta) = f_{y|x}(\beta|\alpha) f_x(\alpha)$$

and

$$f_x(\alpha) = \frac{1}{\sigma_x} f_{z_1}\left(\frac{\alpha - \eta_x}{\sigma_x}\right),$$

we may apply (5.93) to obtain

$$f_{y|x}(\beta|\alpha) = \frac{1}{\sigma_y} f_{z_2|z_1}\left(\frac{\beta - \eta_y}{\sigma_y} \middle| \frac{\alpha - \eta_x}{\sigma_x}\right). \tag{5.94}$$

Substituting (5.90) and (5.87) into (5.93) and (5.94) we find

$$f_{x,y}(\alpha, \beta) = \frac{\exp\left(-\frac{1}{2(1-\rho^2)}\left(\frac{(\alpha-\eta_x)^2}{\sigma_x^2} - \frac{2\rho(\alpha-\eta_x)(\beta-\eta_y)}{\sigma_x \sigma_y} + \frac{(\beta-\eta_y)^2}{\sigma_y^2}\right)\right)}{2\pi \sigma_x \sigma_y (1-\rho^2)^{1/2}} \tag{5.95}$$

and

$$f_{y|x}(\beta|\alpha) = \frac{\exp\left(-\frac{\left(\beta - \eta_y - \rho \sigma_y \frac{\alpha - \eta_x}{\sigma_x}\right)^2}{2(1-\rho^2)\sigma_y^2}\right)}{\sqrt{2\pi \sigma_y^2 (1-\rho^2)}}. \tag{5.96}$$

It follows that

$$E(y|x) = \eta_y + \rho\sigma_y \frac{x - \eta_x}{\sigma_x} \qquad (5.97)$$

and

$$\sigma_{y|x}^2 = \sigma_y^2(1 - \rho^2). \qquad (5.98)$$

By interchanging x with y and α with β,

$$f_{x|y}(\alpha|\beta) = \frac{\exp\left(-\frac{\left(\alpha - \eta_x - \rho\sigma_x \frac{\beta - \eta_y}{\sigma_y}\right)^2}{2(1-\rho^2)\sigma_x^2}\right)}{\sqrt{2\pi\sigma_x^2(1-\rho^2)}}, \qquad (5.99)$$

$$E(x|y) = \eta_x + \rho\sigma_x \frac{y - \eta_y}{\sigma_y}, \qquad (5.100)$$

and

$$\sigma_{x|y}^2 = \sigma_x^2(1 - \rho^2). \qquad (5.101)$$

A three-dimensional plot of a bivariate Gaussian PDF is shown in Figure 5.11.

The bivariate characteristic function for x and y is easily obtained as follows. Since x and y are jointly Gaussian, the RV $t_1 x + t_2 y$ is a univariate Gaussian RV:

$$t_1 x + t_2 y \sim G\left(t_1\eta_x + t_2\eta_y, t_1^2\sigma_x^2 + 2t_1 t_2 \sigma_{x,y} + t_2^2\sigma_y^2\right).$$

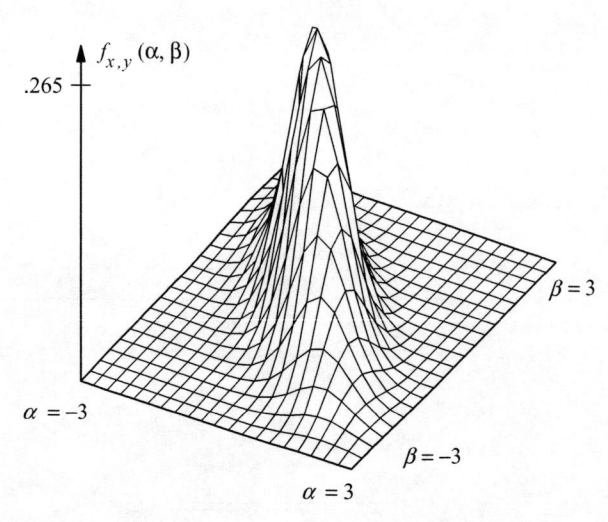

FIGURE 5.11: Bivariate Gaussian PDF $f_{x,y}(\alpha, \beta)$ with $\sigma_x = \sigma_y = 1$, $\eta_x = \eta_y = 0$, and $\rho = -0.8$.

Consequently, the joint characteristic function for x and y is

$$\phi_{x,y}(t_1, t_2) = e^{-\frac{1}{2}(t_1^2\sigma_x^2 + 2t_1t_2\sigma_{x,y} + t_2^2\sigma_y^2)} e^{jt_1\eta_x + jt_2\eta_y}, \quad (5.102)$$

which is valid for all $\sigma_{x,y}$, σ_x and σ_y.

We now consider some special cases of the bivariate Gaussian PDF. If $\rho = 0$ then (from (5.95))

$$f_{x,y}(\alpha, \beta) = f_x(\alpha) f_y(\beta); \quad (5.103)$$

i.e., RVs x and y are independent.

As $\rho \to \pm 1$, from (5.97) and (5.98) we find

$$E(y|x) \to \eta_y \pm \sigma_y \frac{x - \eta_x}{\sigma_x}$$

and $\sigma_{y|x}^2 \to 0$. Hence,

$$y \to \eta_y \pm \sigma_y \frac{x - \eta_x}{\sigma_x}$$

in probability[1]. We conclude that

$$f_{x,y}(\alpha, \beta) = f_x(\alpha) \delta\left(\beta - \eta_y \pm \sigma_y \frac{\alpha - \eta_x}{\sigma_x}\right) \quad (5.104)$$

for $\rho = \pm 1$. Interchanging the roles of x and y we find that the joint PDF for x and y may also be written as

$$f_{x,y}(\alpha, \beta) = f_y(\beta) \delta\left(\alpha - \eta_x \pm \sigma_x \frac{\beta - \eta_y}{\sigma_y}\right) \quad (5.105)$$

when $\rho = \pm 1$. These results can also be obtained "directly" from the joint characteristic function for x and y.

A very special property of jointly Gaussian RVs is presented in the following theorem.

Theorem 5.6.1. *The jointly Gaussian RVs x and y are independent iff $\rho_{x,y} = 0$.*

Proof. We showed previously that if x and y are independent, then $\rho_{x,y} = 0$.
Suppose that $\rho = \rho_{x,y} = 0$. Then $f_{y|x}(\beta|\alpha) = f_y(\beta)$. ∎

Example 5.6.1. *Let x and y be jointly Gaussian with zero means, $\sigma_x^2 = \sigma_y^2 = 1$, and $\rho \neq \pm 1$. Find constants a and b such that $v = ax + by \sim G(0, 1)$ and such that v and x are independent.*

---

[1] As the variance of a RV decreases to zero, the probability that the RV deviates from its mean by more than an arbitrarily small fixed amount approaches zero. This is an application of the Chebyshev Inequality.

Solution. We have $E(v) = 0$. We require

$$\sigma_v^2 = a^2 + b^2 + 2ab\rho_{x,y}^2 = 1$$

and

$$E(vx) = a + b\rho_{x,y} = 0.$$

Hence $a = -b\rho_{x,y}$ and $b^2 = 1/(1 - \rho_{x,y}^2)$, so that

$$v = \frac{y - \rho_{x,y}x}{\sqrt{1 - \rho_{x,y}^2}}$$

is independent of x and $\sigma_v^2 = 1$. ∎

5.6.1 Constant Contours

Returning to the normalized jointly Gaussian RVs z_1 and z_2, we now investigate the shape of the joint PDF $f_{z_1,z_2}(\alpha, \beta)$ by finding the locus of points where the PDF is constant. We assume that $|\rho| < 1$. By inspection of (5.90), we find that $f_{z_1,z_2}(\alpha, \beta)$ is constant for α and β satisfying

$$\alpha^2 - 2\rho\alpha\beta + \beta^2 = c^2, \tag{5.106}$$

where c is a positive constant.

If $\rho = 0$ the contours where the joint PDF is constant is a circle of radius c centered at the origin.

Along the line $\beta = q\alpha$ we find that

$$\alpha^2(1 - 2\rho q + q^2) = c^2 \tag{5.107}$$

so that the constant contours are parameterized by

$$\alpha = \frac{\pm c}{\sqrt{1 - 2\rho q + q^2}}, \tag{5.108}$$

and

$$\beta = \frac{\pm cq}{\sqrt{1 - 2\rho q + q^2}}. \tag{5.109}$$

The square of the distance from a point (α, β) on the contour to the origin is given by

$$d^2(q) = \alpha^2 + \beta^2 = \frac{c^2(1 + q^2)}{1 - 2\rho q + q^2}. \tag{5.110}$$

Differentiating, we find that $d^2(q)$ attains its extremal values at $q = \pm 1$. Thus, the line $\beta = \alpha$ intersects the constant contour at

$$\pm \beta = \alpha = \frac{\pm c}{\sqrt{2(1-\rho)}}. \tag{5.111}$$

Similarly, the line $\beta = -\alpha$, intersects the constant contour at

$$\pm \beta = -\alpha = \frac{\pm c}{\sqrt{2(1-\rho)}}. \tag{5.112}$$

Consider the rotated coordinates $\alpha' = (\alpha + \beta)/\sqrt{2}$ and $\beta' = (\beta - \alpha)/\sqrt{2}$, so that

$$\frac{\alpha' + \beta'}{\sqrt{2}} = \beta \tag{5.113}$$

and

$$\frac{\alpha' - \beta'}{\sqrt{2}} = \alpha. \tag{5.114}$$

The rotated coordinate system is a rotation by $\pi/4$ counterclockwise. Thus

$$\alpha^2 - 2\rho\alpha\beta + \beta^2 = c^2 \tag{5.115}$$

is transformed into

$$\frac{\alpha'^2}{1+\rho} + \frac{\beta'^2}{1-\rho} = \frac{c^2}{1-\rho^2}. \tag{5.116}$$

The above equation represents an ellipse with major axis length $2c/\sqrt{1-|\rho|}$ and minor axis length $2c/\sqrt{1+|\rho|}$. In the $\alpha - \beta$ plane, the major and minor axes of the ellipse are along the lines $\beta = \pm\alpha$.

From (5.93), the constant contours for $f_{x,y}(\alpha, \beta)$ are solutions to

$$\left(\frac{\alpha - \eta_x}{\sigma_x}\right)^2 - 2\rho\left(\frac{\alpha - \eta_x}{\sigma_x}\right)\left(\frac{\beta - \eta_y}{\sigma_y}\right) + \left(\frac{\beta - \eta_y}{\sigma_y}\right)^2 = c^2. \tag{5.117}$$

Using the transformation

$$\alpha' = \frac{1}{\sqrt{2}}\left(\frac{\alpha - \eta_x}{\sigma_x} + \frac{\beta - \eta_y}{\sigma_y}\right), \quad \beta' = \frac{1}{\sqrt{2}}\left(\frac{\beta - \eta_y}{\sigma_y} - \frac{\alpha - \eta_x}{\sigma_x}\right) \tag{5.118}$$

transforms the constant contour to (5.116). With $\alpha' = 0$ we find that one axis is along

$$\frac{\alpha - \eta_x}{\sigma_x} = -\frac{\beta - \eta_y}{\sigma_y}$$

with endpoints at

$$\alpha = \frac{\pm c\sigma_x}{\sqrt{2}\sqrt{1+\rho}} + \eta_x, \quad \beta = \frac{\pm c\sigma_y}{\sqrt{2}\sqrt{1+\rho}} + \eta_y;$$

the length of this axis in the $\alpha - \beta$ plane is

$$\sqrt{2}c\sqrt{\frac{\sigma_x^2 + \sigma_y^2}{1+\rho}}.$$

With $\beta' = 0$ we find that the other axis is along

$$\frac{\alpha - \eta_x}{\sigma_x} = \frac{\beta - \eta_y}{\sigma_y}$$

with endpoints at

$$\alpha = \frac{\pm c\sigma_x}{\sqrt{2}\sqrt{1-\rho}} + \eta_x, \quad \beta = \frac{\pm c\sigma_y}{\sqrt{2}\sqrt{1-\rho}} + \eta_y;$$

the length of this axis in the $\alpha - \beta$ plane is

$$\sqrt{2}c\sqrt{\frac{\sigma_x^2 + \sigma_y^2}{1-\rho}}.$$

Points on this ellipse in the $\alpha - \beta$ plane satisfy (5.117); the value of the joint PDF $f_{x,y}$ on this curve is

$$\frac{1}{2\pi\sigma_x\sigma_y\sqrt{1-\rho^2}} \exp\left(-\frac{c^2}{2(1-\rho^2)}\right). \tag{5.119}$$

A further transformation

$$\alpha'' = \frac{\alpha'}{\sqrt{1+\rho}}, \quad \beta'' = \frac{\beta'}{\sqrt{1-\rho}}$$

transforms the ellipse in the $\alpha' - \beta'$ plane to a circle in the $\alpha'' - \beta''$ plane:

$$\alpha''^2 + \beta''^2 = \frac{c^2}{1-\rho^2}.$$

This transformation provides a straightforward way to compute the probability that the joint Gaussian RVs x and y lie within the region bounded by the ellipse specified by (5.117). Letting A denote the region bounded by the ellipse in the $\alpha - \beta$ plane and A'' denote the image (a circle)

STANDARD PROBABILITY DISTRIBUTIONS

in the $\alpha'' - \beta''$ plane, we have

$$\iint_A f_{x,y}(\alpha,\beta)\,d\alpha\,d\beta = \iint \frac{1}{2\pi\sigma_x\sigma_y\sqrt{1-\rho^2}} \frac{e^{-\frac{1}{2}(\alpha''^2+\beta''^2)}}{|J(\alpha,\beta)|}\,d\alpha''\,d\beta'',$$

where the Jacobian of the transformation is

$$J(\alpha,\beta) = \begin{vmatrix} \dfrac{\partial \alpha''}{\partial \alpha} & \dfrac{\partial \alpha''}{\partial \beta} \\ \dfrac{\partial \beta''}{\partial \alpha} & \dfrac{\partial \beta''}{\partial \beta} \end{vmatrix}.$$

Computing the indicated derivatives, we have

$$J(\alpha,\beta) = \begin{vmatrix} \dfrac{1}{\sigma_x\sqrt{2}\sqrt{1+\rho}} & \dfrac{1}{\sigma_y\sqrt{2}\sqrt{1+\rho}} \\ \dfrac{-1}{\sigma_x\sqrt{2}\sqrt{1-\rho}} & \dfrac{1}{\sigma_y\sqrt{2}\sqrt{1-\rho}} \end{vmatrix},$$

so that

$$J(\alpha,\beta) = \frac{1}{\sigma_x\sigma_y\sqrt{1-\rho^2}}.$$

Substituting and transforming to polar coordinates, we find

$$\iint_A f_{x,y}(\alpha,\beta)\,d\alpha\,d\beta = \iint_{A''} \frac{1}{2\pi} e^{-\frac{1}{2}(\alpha''^2+\beta''^2)}\,d\alpha''\,d\beta''$$

$$= \frac{1}{2\pi} \int_0^{2\pi} \int_0^{c/\sqrt{1-\rho^2}} r e^{-\frac{1}{2}r^2}\,dr\,d\theta$$

$$= \int_0^{c^2/(2-2\rho^2)} e^{-u}\,du$$

$$= 1 - e^{-c^2/(2-2\rho^2)}.$$

This bivariate Gaussian probability computation is one of the few which is "easily" accomplished. Additional techniques for treating these computations are given in [1, pp. 956–958].

Drill Problem 5.6.1. *Given that x and y are jointly distributed Gaussian random variables with $E(y|x) = 2 + 1.5x$, $E(x|y) = 7/6 + y/6$, and $\sigma_{x|y}^2 = 0.75$. Determine: (a) η_x, (b) η_y, (c) σ_x^2, (d) σ_y^2, and (e) $\rho_{x,y}$.*

Answers: 0.5, 1, 9, 2, 5.

Drill Problem 5.6.2. *Random variables x and y are jointly Gaussian with $\eta_x = -2$, $\eta_y = 3$, $\sigma_x^2 = 21$, $\sigma_y^2 = 31$, and $\rho = -0.3394$. With $c^2 = 0.2212$ in (154), find: (a) the smallest angle that either the minor or major axis makes with the positive α axis in the $\alpha - \beta$ plane, (b) the length of the minor axis, (c) the length of the major axis.*

Answers: 3, 2, 30°.

Drill Problem 5.6.3. *Random variables x and y are jointly Gaussian with $\eta_x = -2$, $\eta_y = 3$, $\sigma_x^2 = 21$, $\sigma_y^2 = 31$, and $\rho = -0.3394$. Find: (a) $E(y \mid x = 0)$, (b) $P(1 < y \leq 10 \mid x = 0)$, (c) $P(-1 < x < 7)$.*

Answers: 0.5212, 0.3889, 2.1753.

5.7 SUMMARY

This chapter introduces certain probability distributions commonly encountered in biomedical engineering. Special emphasis is placed on the exponential, Poisson and Gaussian distributions. Important approximations to the Bernoulli PMF and Gaussian CDF are developed.

Bernoulli event probabilities may be approximated by the Poisson PMF when $np < 10$ or by the Gaussian PDF when $npq > 3$. For the Poisson approximation use $\eta = np$. For the Gaussian approximation use $\eta = np$ and $\sigma^2 = npq$.

Many important properties of jointly Gaussian random variables are presented.

Drill Problem 5.7.1. *The length of time William Smith plays a video game is given by random variable x distributed exponentially with a mean of four minutes. His play during each game is independent from all other games. Determine: (a) the probability that William is still playing after four minutes, (b) the probability that, out of five games, he has played at least one game for more than four minutes.*

Answers: exp(−1), 0.899.

5.8 PROBLEMS

1. Assume x is a Bernoulli random variable. Determine $P(x \leq 3)$ using the Bernoulli CDF table if: (a) $n = 5$, $p = 0.1$; (b) $n = 10$, $p = 0.1$; (c) $n = 20$, $p = 0.1$; (d) $n = 5$, $p = 0.3$; (e) $n = 10$, $p = 0.3$; (f) $n = 20$, $p = 0.3$; (g) $n = 5$, $p = 0.6$; (h) $n = 10$, $p = 0.6$; (i) $n = 20$, $p = 0.6$.

2. Suppose you are playing a game with a friend in which you roll a die 10 times. If the die comes up with an even number, your friend gives you a dollar and if the die comes up with an odd number you give your friend a dollar. Unfortunately, the die is loaded

so that a 1 or a 3 are three times as likely to occur as a 2, a 4, a 5 or a 6. Determine: (a) how many dollars your friend can expect to win in this game; (b) the probability of your friend winning more than 4 dollars.

3. The probability that a basketball player makes a basket is 0.4. If he makes 10 attempts, what is the probability he will make: (a) at least 4 baskets; (b) 4 baskets; (c) from 7 to 9 baskets; (d) less than 2 baskets; (e) the expected number of baskets.

4. The probability that Professor Rensselaer bowls a strike is 0.2. Determine the probability that: (a) 3 of the next 20 rolls are strikes; (b) at least 4 of the next 20 rolls are strikes; (c) from 3 to 7 of the next 20 rolls are strikes. (d) She is to keep rolling the ball until she gets a strike. Determine the probability it will take more than 5 rolls. Determine the: (e) expected number of strikes in 20 rolls; (f) variance for the number of strikes in 20 rolls; (g) standard deviation for the number of strikes in 20 rolls.

5. The probability of a man hitting a target is 0.3. (a) If he tries 15 times to hit the target, what is the probability of him hitting it at least 5 but less than 10 times? (b) What is the average number of hits in 30 tries? (c) What is the probability of him getting exactly the average number of hits in 30 tries? (d) How many times must the man try to hit the target if he wants the probability of hitting it to be at least 2/3? (e) What is the probability that no more than three tries are required to hit the target for the first time?

6. In Junior Bioinstrumentation Lab, one experiment introduces students to the transistor. Each student is given only one transistor to use. The probability of a student destroying a transistor is 0.7. One lab class has 5 students and they will perform this experiment next week. Let random variable x show the possible numbers of students who destroy transistors. (a) Sketch the PMF for x. Determine: (b) the expected number of destroyed transistors, (c) the probability that fewer than 2 transistors are destroyed.

7. On a frosty January morning in Fargo, North Dakota, the probability that a car parked outside will start is 0.6. (a) If we take a sample of 20 cars, what is the probability that exactly 12 cars will start and 8 will not? (b) What is the probability that the number of cars starting out of 20 is between 9 and 15.

8. Consider Problem 7. If there are 20,000 cars to be started, find the probability that: (a) at least 12,100 will start; (b) exactly 12,000 will start; (c) the number starting is between 11,900 and 12,150; (d) the number starting is less than 12,500.

9. A dart player has found that the probability of hitting the dart board in any one throw is 0.2. How many times must he throw the dart so that the probability of hitting the dart board is at least 0.6?

10. Let random variable x be Bernoulli with $n = 15$ and $p = 0.4$. Determine $E(x^2)$.

11. Suppose x is a Bernoulli random variable with $\eta = 10$ and $\sigma^2 = 10/3$. Determine: (a) q, (b) n, (c) p.

12. An electronics manufacturer is evaluating its quality control program. The current procedure is to take a sample of 5 from 1000 and pass the shipment if not more than 1 component is found defective. What proportion of 20% defective components will be shipped?

13. Repeat Problem 1, when appropriate, using the Poisson approximation to the Bernoulli PMF.

14. A certain intersection averages 3 traffic accidents per week. What is the probability that more than 2 accidents will occur during any given week?

15. Suppose that on the average, a student makes 6 mistakes per test. Determine the probability that the student makes: (a) at least 1 mistake; (b) from 3 to 5 mistakes; (c) exactly 2 mistakes; (d) more than the expected number of mistakes.

16. On the average, Professor Rensselaer gives 11 quizzes per quarter in Introduction to Random Processes. Determine the probability that: (a) from 8 to 12 quizzes are given during the quarter; (b) exactly 11 quizzes are given during the quarter; (c) at least 10 quizzes are given during the quarter; (d) at most 9 quizzes are given during the quarter.

17. Suppose a typist makes an average of 30 mistakes per page. (a) If you give him a one page letter to type, what is the probability that he makes exactly 30 mistakes? (b) The typist decides to take typing lessons, and, after the lessons, he averages 5 mistakes per page. You give him another one page letter to type. What is the probability of him making fewer than 5 mistakes. (c) With the 5 mistakes per page average, what is the probability of him making fewer than 50 mistakes in a 25 page report?

18. On the average, a sample of radioactive material emits 20 alpha particles per minute. What is the probability of 10 alpha particles being emitted in: (a) 1 min, (b) 10 min? (c) Many years later, the material averages 6 alpha particles emitted per minute. What is the probability of at least 6 alpha particles being emitted in 1 min?

19. At Fargo Polytechnic Institute (FPI), a student may take a course as many times as desired. Suppose the average number of times a student takes Introduction to Random Processes is 1.5. (Professor Rensselaer, the course instructor, thinks so many students repeat the course because they enjoy it so much.) (a) Determine the probability that a student takes the course more than once. (b) The academic vice-president of FPI wants to ensure that on the average, 80% of the students take the course at most one time. To what value should the mean be adjusted to ensure this?

STANDARD PROBABILITY DISTRIBUTIONS   39

20. Suppose 1% of the transistors in a box are defective. Determine the probability that there are: (a) 3 defective transistors in a sample of 200 transistors; (b) more than 15 defective transistors in a sample of 1000 transistors; (c) 0 defective transistors in a sample of 20 transistors.

21. A perfect car is assembled with a probability of 2×10^{-5}. If 15,000 cars are produced in a month, what is the probability that none are perfect?

22. FPI admits only 1000 freshmen per year. The probability that a student will major in Bioengineering is 0.01. Determine the probability that fewer than 9 students major in Bioengineering.

23. (a) Every time a carpenter pounds in a nail, the probability that he hits his thumb is 0.002. If in building a house he pounds 1250 nails, what is the probability of him hitting his thumb at least once while working on the house? (b) If he takes five extra minutes off every time he hits his thumb, how many extra minutes can he expect to take off in building a house with 3000 nails?

24. The manufacturer of Leaping Lizards, a bran cereal with milk expanding (exploding) marshmallow lizards, wants to ensure that on the average, 95% of the spoonfuls will each have at least one lizard. Assuming that the lizards are randomly distributed in the cereal box, to what value should the mean of the lizards per spoonful be set at to ensure this?

25. The distribution for the number of students seeking advising help from Professor Rensselaer during any particular day is given by

$$P(x = k) = \frac{3^k e^{-3}}{k!}, \qquad k = 0, 1, \ldots.$$

The PDF for the time interval between students seeking help for Introduction to Random Processes from Professor Rensselaer during any particular day is given by

$$f_t(\tau) = e^{-\tau} u(\tau).$$

If random variable z equals the total number of students Professor Rensselaer helps each day, determine: (a) $E(z)$, (b) σ_z.

26. This year, on its anniversary day, a computer store is going to run an advertising campaign in which the employees will telephone 5840 people selected at random from the population of North America. The caller will ask the person answering the phone if it's his or her birthday. If it is, then that lucky person will be mailed a brand new programmable calculator. Otherwise, that person will get nothing. Assuming that

the person answering the phone won't lie and that there is no such thing as leap year, find the probability that: (a) the computer store mails out exactly 16 calculators, (b) the computer store mails out from 20 to 40 calculators.

27. Random variable x is uniform between -2 and 3. Event $A = \{0 < x \leq 2\}$ and $B = \{-1 < x \leq 0\} \cup \{1 < x \leq 2\}$. Find: (a) $P(-1 < x < 0)$, (b) η_x, (c) σ_x, (d) $f_{x|A}(\alpha|A)$, (e) $F_{x|A}(\alpha|A)$, (f) $f_{x|B}(\alpha|B)$, (g) $F_{x|B}(\alpha|B)$.

28. The time it takes a runner to run a mile is equally likely to lie in an interval from 4.0 to 4.2 min. Determine: (a) the probability it takes the runner exactly 4 min to run a mile, (b) the probability it takes the runner from 4.1 to 4.15 min.

29. Assume x is a standard Gaussian random variable. Using Tables A.9 and A.10, determine: (a) $P(x = 0)$, (b) $P(x < 0)$, (c) $P(x < 0.2)$, (d) $P(-1.583 \leq x < 1.471)$, (e) $P(-2.1 < x \leq -0.5)$, (f) $P(x$ is an integer$)$.

30. Repeat Problem 1, when appropriate, using the Gaussian approximation to the Bernoulli PMF.

31. A light bulb manufacturer distributes light bulbs that have a length of life that is normally distributed with a mean equal to 1200 h and a standard deviation of 40 h. Find the probability that a bulb burns between 1000 and 1300 h.

32. A certain type of resistor has resistance values that are Gaussian distributed with a mean of 50 ohms and a variance of 3. (a) Write the PDF for the resistance value. (b) Find the probability that a particular resistor is within 2 ohms of the mean. (c) Find $P(49 < r < 54)$.

33. Consider Problem 32. If resistances are measured to the nearest ohm, find: (a) the probability that a particular resistor is within 2 ohms of the mean, (b) $P(49 < r < 54)$.

34. A battery manufacturer has found that 8.08% of their batteries last less than 2.3 years and 2.5% of their batteries last more than 3.98 years. Assuming the battery lives are Gaussian distributed, find: (a) the mean, (b) variance.

35. Assume that the scores on an examination are Gaussian distributed with mean 75 and standard deviation 10. Grades are assigned as follows: A: 90–100, B: 80–90, C: 70–80, D: 60–70, and F: below 60. In a class of 25 students, what is the probability that grades will be equally distributed?

36. A certain transistor has a current gain, h, that is Gaussian distributed with a mean of 77 and a variance of 11. Find: (a) $P(h > 74)$, (b) $P(73 < h \leq 80)$, (c) $P(|h - \eta_h| < 3\sigma_h)$.

37. Consider Problem 36. Find the value of d so that the range $77 + d$ covers 95% of the current gains.

38. A 250 question multiple choice final exam is given. Each question has 5 possible answers and only one correct answer. Determine the probability that a student guesses the correct answers for 20–25 of 85 questions about which the student has no knowledge.

39. The average golf score for Professor Rensselaer is 78 with a standard deviation of 3. Assuming a Gaussian distribution for random variable x describing her golf game, determine: (a) $P(x = 78)$, (b) $P(x \leq 78)$, (c) $P(70 < x \leq 80)$, (d) the probability that x is less than 75 if the score is measured to the nearest unit.

40. Suppose a system contains a component whose length is normally distributed with a mean of 2.0 and a standard deviation of 0.2. If 5 of these components are removed from different systems, what is the probability that at least 2 have a length greater than 2.1?

41. A large box contains 10,000 resistors with resistances that are Gaussian distributed. If the average resistance is 1000 ohms with a standard deviation of 200 ohms, how many resistors have resistances that are within 10% of the average?

42. The RV x has PDF
$$f_x(\alpha) = a \exp\left(-\frac{1}{2\sigma^2}(\alpha - \eta)^2\right).$$
(a) Find the constant a. (Hint: assume RV y is independent of x and has PDF $f_y(\beta) = f_x(\beta)$ and evaluate $F_{x,y}(\infty, \infty)$.) (b) Using direct integration, find $E(x)$. (c) Find σ_x^2 using direct integration.

43. Assume x and y are jointly distributed Gaussian random variables with $x \sim G(-2, 4)$, $y \sim G(3, 9)$, and $\rho_{x,y} = 0$. Find: (a) $P(1 < y < 7 \mid x = 0)$, (b) $P(1 < y < 7)$, (c) $P(-1 < x < 1, 1 < y < 7)$.

44. Suppose x and y are jointly distributed Gaussian random variables with $E(y|x) = 2.8 + 0.32x$, $E(x|y) = -1 + 0.5y$, and $\sigma_{y|x} = 3.67$. Determine: (a) η_x, (b) η_y, (c) σ_x, (d) σ_y, (e) $\rho_{x,y}$, (f) $\sigma_{x,y}$.

45. Assume $x \sim G(3, 1)$, $y \sim G(-2, 1)$, and that x and y are jointly Gaussian with $\rho_{x,y} = -0.5$. Draw a sketch of the joint Gaussian contour equation showing the original and the translated-rotated sets of axes.

46. Consider Problem 45. Determine: (a) $E(y|x=0)$, (b) $f_{y|x}(\beta|0)$, (c) $P(0 < y < 4|x=0)$, (d) $P(3 < x < 10)$.

47. Assume x and y are jointly Gaussian with $x \sim G(2, 13)$, $y \sim G(1, 8)$, and $\rho_{x,y} = -5.8835$. (a) Draw a sketch of the constant contour equation for the standardized RVs z_1 and z_2. (b) Using the results of (a), Draw a sketch of the joint Gaussian constant contour for x and y.

48. Consider Problem 47. Determine: (a) $E(y|x=0)$, (b) $f_{y|x}(\beta|0)$, (c) $P(0 < y < 4|x=0)$, (d) $P(3 < x < 10)$.

49. Assume x and y are jointly Gaussian with $x \sim G(-1, 4)$, $y \sim G(1.6, 7)$, and $\rho_{x,y} = 0.378$. (a) Draw a sketch of the constant contour equation for the standardized RVs z_1 and z_2. (b) Using the results of (a), Draw a sketch of the joint Gaussian contour for x and y.

50. Consider Problem 49. Determine: (a) $E(y|x=0)$, (b) $f_{y|x}(\beta|0)$, (c) $P(0 < y < 4|x=0)$, (d) $P(-3 < x < 0)$.

51. A component with an exponential failure rate is 90% reliable at 10,000 h. Determine the number of hours reliable at 95%.

52. Suppose a system has an exponential failure rate in years to failure with $\eta = 2.5$. Determine the number of years reliable at: (a) 90%, (b) 95%, (c) 99%.

53. Consider Problem 52. If 20 of these systems are installed, determine the probability that 10 are operating at the end of 2.3 years.

54. In the circuit shown in Figure 5.12, each of the four components operate independently of one another and have an exponential failure rate (in hours) with $\eta = 10^5$. For successful operation of the circuit, at least two of these components must connect A with B. Determine the probability that the circuit is operating successfully at 10,000 h.

55. The survival rate of individuals with a certain type of cancer is assumed to be exponential with $\eta = 4$ years. Five individuals have this cancer. Determine the probability that at most three will be alive at the end of 2.0433 years.

56. Random variable t is exponential with $\eta = 2$. Determine: (a) $P(t > \eta)$, (b) $f_z(\alpha)$ if $z = t - T$, where T is a constant.

57. William Smith is a varsity wrestler on his high school team. Without exception, if he does not pin his opponent with his trick move, he loses the match on points. William's

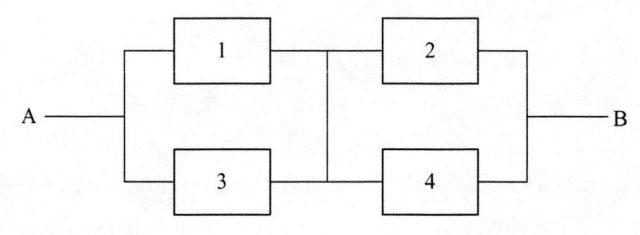

FIGURE 5.12: Circuit for Problem 54.

trick move also prevents him from ever getting pinned. The length of time it takes William to pin his opponent in each period of a wrestling match is given by:

$$\text{period 1}: f_x(\alpha) = 0.4598394 \exp(-0.4598394\alpha)u(\alpha),$$
$$\text{period 2}: f_{x|A}(\alpha|A) = 0.2299197 \exp(-0.2299197\alpha)u(\alpha),$$
$$\text{period 3}: f_{x|A}(\alpha|A) = 0.1149599 \exp(-0.1149599\alpha)u(\alpha),$$

where $A = \{$Smith did not pin his opponent during the previous periods$\}$. Assume each period is 2 min and the match is 3 periods. Determine the probability that William Smith: (a) pins his opponent during the first period: (b) pins his opponent during the second period: (c) pins his opponent during the third period: (d) wins the match.

58. Consider Problem 57. Find the probability that William Smith wins: (a) at least 4 of his first 5 matches, (b) more matches than he is expected to during a 10 match season.

59. The average time between power failures in a Coop utility is once every 1.4 years. Determine: (a) the probability that there will be at least one power failure during the coming year, (b) the probability that there will be at least two power failures during the coming year.

60. Consider Problem 59 statement. Assume that a power failure will last at least 24 h. Suppose Fargo Community Hospital has a backup emergency generator to provide auxilary power during a power failure. Moreover, the emergency generator has an expected time between failures of once every 200 h. What is the probability that the hospital will be without power during the next 24 h?

61. The queue for the cash register at a popular package store near Fargo Polytechnic Institute becomes quite long on Saturdays following football games. On the average, the queue is 6.3 people long. Each customer takes 4 min to check out. Determine: (a) your expected waiting time to make a purchase, (b) the probability that you will have less than four people in the queue ahead of you, (c) the probability that you will have more than five people in the queue ahead of you.

62. Outer Space Adventures, Inc. prints brochures describing their vacation packages as "Unique, Unexpected and Unexplained." The vacations certainly live up to their advertisement. In fact, they are so unexpected that the length of the vacations is random, following an exponential distribution, having an average length of 6 months. Suppose that you have signed up for a vacation trip that starts at the end of this quarter. What is the probability that you will be back home in time for next fall quarter (that is, 9 months later)?

63. A certain brand of light bulbs has an average life-expectancy of 750 h. The failure rate of these light bulbs follows an exponential PDF. Seven-hundred and fifty of these bulbs were put in light fixtures in four rooms. The lights were turned on and left that way for a different length of time in each room as follows:

ROOM	TIME BULBS LEFT ON, HOURS	NUMBER OF BULBS
1	1000	125
2	750	250
3	500	150
4	1500	225

After the specified length of time, the bulbs were taken from the fixtures and placed in a box. If a bulb is selected at random from the box, what is the probability that it is burnt out?

CHAPTER 6

Transformations of Random Variables

Functions of random variables occur frequently in many applications of probability theory. For example, a full wave rectifier circuit produces an output that is the absolute value of the input. The input/output characteristics of many physical devices can be represented by a nonlinear memoryless transformation of the input.

The primary subjects of this chapter are methods for determining the probability distribution of a function of a random variable. We first evaluate the probability distribution of a function of one random variable using the CDF and then the PDF. Next, the probability distribution for a single random variable is determined from a function of two random variables using the CDF. Then, the joint probability distribution is found from a function of two random variables using the joint PDF and the CDF.

6.1 UNIVARIATE CDF TECHNIQUE

This section introduces a method of computing the probability distribution of a function of a random variable using the CDF. We will refer to this method as the CDF technique. The CDF technique is applicable for all functions $z = g(x)$, and for all types of continuous, discrete, and mixed random variables. Of course, we require that the function $z: S \mapsto R^*$, with $z(\zeta) = g(x(\zeta))$, is a random variable on the probability space $(S, \Im, P)$; consequently, we require z to be a measurable function on the measurable space $(S, \Im)$ and $P(z(\zeta) \in \{-\infty, +\infty\}) = 0$.

The ease of use of the CDF technique depends critically on the functional form of $g(x)$. To make the CDF technique easier to understand, we start the discussion of computing the probability distribution of $z = g(x)$ with the simplest case, a continuous monotonic function g. (Recall that if g is a monotonic function then a one-to-one correspondence between $g(x)$ and x exists.) Then, the difficulties associated with computing the probability distribution of $z = g(x)$ are investigated when the restrictions on $g(x)$ are relaxed.

6.1.1 CDF Technique with Monotonic Functions

Consider the problem where the CDF F_x is known for the RV x, and we wish to find the CDF for random variable $z = g(x)$. Proceeding from the definition of the CDF for z, we have for a monotonic increasing function $g(x)$

$$F_z(\gamma) = P(z = g(x) \leq \gamma) = P(x \leq g^{-1}(\gamma)) = F_x(g^{-1}(\gamma)), \qquad (6.1)$$

where $g^{-1}(\gamma)$ is the value of α for which $g(\alpha) = \gamma$. As (6.1) indicates, the CDF of random variable z is written in terms of $F_x(\alpha)$, with the argument α replaced by $g^{-1}(\gamma)$.

Similarly, if $z = g(x)$ and g is monotone decreasing, then

$$F_z(\gamma) = P(z = g(x) \leq \gamma) = P(x \geq g^{-1}(\gamma)) = 1 - F_x(g^{-1}(\gamma)^-). \qquad (6.2)$$

The following example illustrates this technique.

Example 6.1.1. *Random variable x is uniformly distributed in the interval 0 to 4. Find the CDF for random variable $z = 2x + 1$.*

Solution. Since random variable x is uniformly distributed, the CDF of x is

$$F_x(\alpha) = \begin{cases} 0, & \alpha < 0 \\ \alpha/4, & 0 \leq \alpha < 4 \\ 1, & 4 \leq \alpha. \end{cases}$$

Letting $g(x) = 2x + 1$, we see that g is monotone increasing and that $g^{-1}(\gamma) = (\gamma - 1)/2$. Applying (6.1), the CDF for z is given by

$$F_z(\gamma) = F_x\left(\frac{\gamma - 1}{2}\right) = \begin{cases} 0, & (\gamma - 1)/2 < 0 \\ (\gamma - 1)/8, & 0 \leq (\gamma - 1)/2 < 4 \\ 1, & 4 \leq (\gamma - 1)/2. \end{cases}$$

Simplifying, we obtain

$$F_z(\gamma) = \begin{cases} 0, & \gamma < 1 \\ (\gamma - 1)/8, & 1 \leq \gamma < 9 \\ 1, & 9 \leq \gamma, \end{cases}$$

which is also a uniform distribution. ∎

6.1.2 CDF Technique with Arbitrary Functions

In general, the relationship between x and z can take on any form, including discontinuities. Additionally, the function does not have to be monotonic, more than one solution of $z = g(x)$ can exist—resulting in a many-to-one mapping from x to z. In general, the only requirement on g is that $z = g(x)$ be a random variable. In this general case, $F_z(\gamma)$ is no longer found by simple substitution. In fact, under these conditions it is impossible to write a general expression for $F_z(\gamma)$ using the CDF technique. However, this case is conceptually no more difficult than

the previous case, and involves only careful book keeping.
Let
$$A(\gamma) = \{x : g(x) \leq \gamma\}. \qquad (6.3)$$
Note that $A(\gamma) = g^{-1}((-\infty, \gamma])$. Then
$$F_z(\gamma) = P(g(x) \leq \gamma) = P(x \in A(\gamma)). \qquad (6.4)$$
Partition $A(\gamma)$ into disjoint intervals $\{A_i(\gamma) : i = 1, 2, \ldots\}$ so that
$$A(\gamma) = \bigcup_{i=1}^{\infty} A_i(\gamma). \qquad (6.5)$$
Note that the intervals as well as the number of nonempty intervals depends on γ. Since the A_i's are disjoint,
$$F_z(\gamma) = \sum_{i=1}^{\infty} P(x \in A_i(\gamma)). \qquad (6.6)$$
The above probabilities are easily found from the CDF F_x. If interval $A_i(\gamma)$ is of the form
$$A_i(\gamma) = (a_i(\gamma), b_i(\gamma)], \qquad (6.7)$$
then
$$P(x \in A_i(\gamma)) = F_x(b_i(\gamma)) - F_x(a_i(\gamma)). \qquad (6.8)$$
Similarly, if interval $A_i(\gamma)$ is of the form
$$A_i(\gamma) = [a_i(\gamma), b_i(\gamma)], \qquad (6.9)$$
then
$$P(x \in A_i(\gamma)) = F_x(b_i(\gamma)) - F_x(a_i(\gamma)^-). \qquad (6.10)$$
The success of this method clearly depends on our ability to partition $A(\gamma)$ into disjoint intervals. Using this method, any function g and CDF F_x is amenable to a solution for $F_z(\gamma)$. The following examples illustrate various aspects of this technique.

Example 6.1.2. *Random variable x has the CDF*
$$F_x(\alpha) = \begin{cases} 0, & \alpha < -1 \\ (3\alpha - \alpha^3 + 2)/4, & -1 \leq \alpha < 1 \\ 1, & 1 \leq \alpha. \end{cases}$$
Find the CDF for the RV $z = x^2$.

48   ADVANCED PROBABILITY THEORY FOR BIOMEDICAL ENGINEERS

Solution. Letting $g(x) = x^2$, we find

$$A(\gamma) = g^{-1}((-\infty, \gamma]) = \begin{cases} \emptyset, & \gamma < 0 \\ [-\sqrt{\gamma}, \sqrt{\gamma}], & \gamma \geq 0. \end{cases}$$

so that

$$F_z(\gamma) = F_x(\sqrt{\gamma}) - F_x((-\sqrt{\gamma})^-).$$

Noting that $F_x(\alpha)$ is continuous and has the same functional form for $-1 < \alpha < 1$, we obtain

$$F_z(\gamma) = \begin{cases} 0, & \gamma < 0 \\ (3\sqrt{\gamma} - (\sqrt{\gamma})^3)/2, & 0 \leq \gamma < 1 \\ 1 & 1 \leq \gamma. \end{cases}$$

∎

Example 6.1.3. *Random variable x is uniformly distributed in the interval −3 to 3. Random variable z is defined by*

$$z = g(x) = \begin{cases} -1, & x < -2 \\ 3x + 5, & -2 \leq x < -1 \\ -3x - 1, & -1 \leq x < 0 \\ 3x - 1, & 0 \leq x < 1 \\ 2, & 1 \leq x. \end{cases}$$

Find $F_z(\gamma)$.

Solution. Plots for this example are given in Figure 6.1. The CDF for random variable x is

$$F_x(\alpha) = \begin{cases} 0, & \alpha < -3 \\ (\alpha + 3)/6, & -3 \leq \alpha < 3 \\ 1, & 3 \leq \alpha. \end{cases}$$

Let $A(\gamma) = g^{-1}((-\infty, \infty))$. Referring to Figure 6.1 we find

$$A(\gamma) = \begin{cases} \emptyset, & \gamma < -1 \\ \left(-\infty, \dfrac{\gamma - 5}{3}\right] \cup \left[\dfrac{-\gamma - 1}{3}, \dfrac{\gamma + 1}{3}\right], & -1 \leq \gamma < 2 \\ R & 2 \leq \gamma. \end{cases}$$

Consequently,

$$F_z(\gamma) = \begin{cases} 0, & \gamma < -1 \\ F_x\left(\dfrac{\gamma - 5}{3}\right) + F_x\left(\dfrac{\gamma + 1}{3}\right) - F_x\left(\left(\dfrac{-\gamma - 1}{3}\right)^-\right), & -1 \leq \gamma < 2 \\ 1 & 2 \leq \gamma. \end{cases}$$

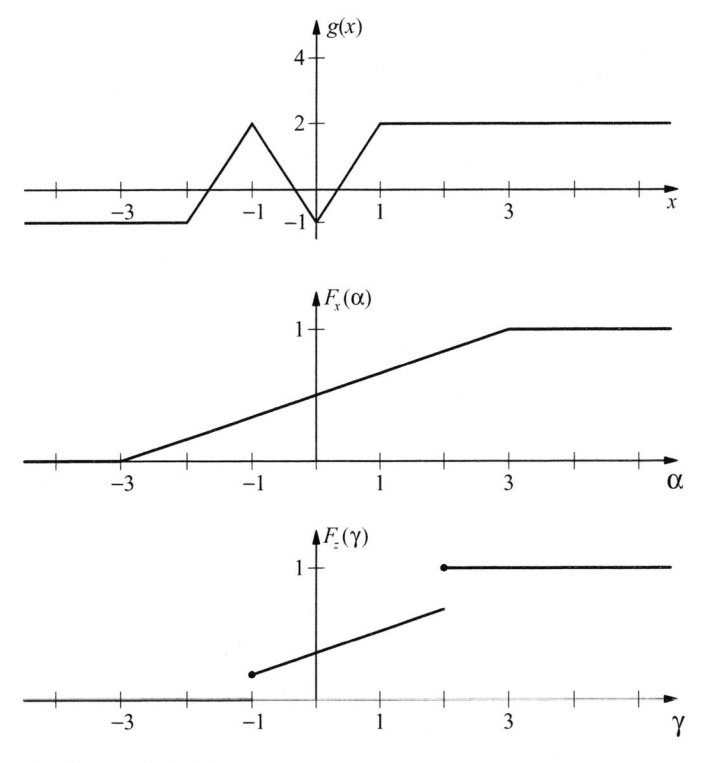

FIGURE 6.1: Plots for Example 6.1.3.

Substituting, we obtain

$$F_z(\gamma) = \begin{cases} 0, & \gamma < -1 \\ \dfrac{1}{6}\left(\dfrac{\gamma-5}{3} + 3 + \dfrac{\gamma+1}{3} - \dfrac{-\gamma-1}{3}\right) = \dfrac{\gamma+2}{6}, & -1 \leq \gamma < 2 \\ 1 & 2 \leq \gamma. \end{cases}$$

Note that $F_z(\gamma)$ has jumps at $\gamma = -1$ and at $\gamma = 2$. ∎

Whenever random variable x is continuous and $g(x)$ is constant over some interval or intervals, then random variable z can be continuous, discrete or mixed, dependent on the CDF for random variable x. As presented in the previous example, random variable z is mixed due to the constant value of $g(x)$ in the intervals $-3 \leq x < -2$ and $1 \leq x < 3$. In fact, z is a mixed random variable whenever $g(\alpha)$ is constant in an interval where $f_x(\alpha) \neq 0$. This results in a jump in F_z and an impulse function in f_z. Moreover, $z = g(x)$ is a discrete random variable if $g(\alpha)$ changes values only on intervals where $f_x(\alpha) = 0$. Random variable z is continuous if x is continuous and $g(x)$ is not equal to a constant over any interval where $f_x(\alpha) \neq 0$.

50 ADVANCED PROBABILITY THEORY FOR BIOMEDICAL ENGINEERS

Example 6.1.4. *Random variable x has the PDF*

$$f_x(\alpha) = \begin{cases} (1+\alpha^2)/6, & -1 < \alpha < 2 \\ 0, & \text{otherwise.} \end{cases}$$

Find the PDF of random variable z defined by

$$z = g(x) = \begin{cases} x-1, & x \leq 0 \\ 0, & 0 < x \leq 0.5 \\ 1, & 0.5 < x. \end{cases}$$

Solution. To find f_z, we evaluate F_z first, then differentiate this result. The CDF for random variable x is

$$F_x(\alpha) = \begin{cases} 0, & \alpha < -1 \\ (\alpha^3 + 3\alpha + 4)/18, & -1 \leq \alpha < 2 \\ 1, & 2 \leq \alpha. \end{cases}$$

Figure 6.2 shows a plot of $g(x)$. With the aid of Figure 6.2, we find

$$A(\gamma) = \{x : g(x) \leq \gamma\} = \begin{cases} (-\infty, \gamma+1], & \gamma \leq -1 \\ (-\infty, 0], & -1 \leq \gamma < 0 \\ (-\infty, 0.5], & 0 \leq \gamma < 1 \\ (-\infty, \infty), & 1 \leq \gamma. \end{cases}$$

Consequently,

$$F_z(\gamma) = \begin{cases} F_x(\gamma+1), & \gamma \leq -1 \\ F_x(0), & -1 \leq \gamma < 0 \\ F_x(0.5), & 0 \leq \gamma < 1 \\ 1, & 1 \leq \gamma. \end{cases}$$

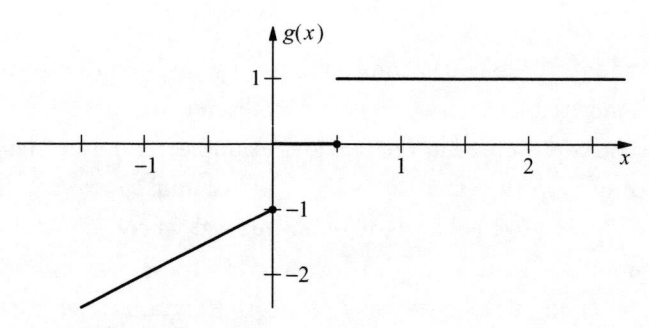

FIGURE 6.2: Transformation for Example 6.1.4.

Substituting,

$$F_z(\gamma) = \begin{cases} 0, & \gamma < -2 \\ ((\gamma+1)^3 + 3\gamma + 7)/18, & -2 \leq \gamma < -1 \\ 2/9, & -1 \leq \gamma < 0 \\ 5/16, & 0 \leq \gamma < 1 \\ 1, & 1 \leq \gamma. \end{cases}$$

Note that $F_z(\gamma)$ has jumps at $\gamma = 0$ and $\gamma = 1$ of heights 13/144 and 11/16, respectively. Differentiating F_z,

$$f_z(\gamma) = \frac{3\gamma^2 + 6\gamma + 6}{18}(u(\gamma+2) - u(\gamma+1)) + \frac{13}{144}\delta(\gamma) + \frac{11}{16}\delta(\gamma-1).$$ ■

Example 6.1.5. *Random variable x is uniformly distributed in the interval from 0 to 10. Find the CDF for random variable $z = g(x) = -\ln(x)$.*

Solution. The CDF for x is

$$F_x(\alpha) = \begin{cases} 0, & \alpha < 0 \\ \alpha/10, & 0 \leq \alpha < 10 \\ 1, & 10 \leq \alpha. \end{cases}$$

For $\gamma > 0$, we find

$$A(\gamma) = \{x : -\ln(x) \leq \gamma\} = (e^{-\gamma}, \infty),$$

so that $F_z(\gamma) = 1 - F_x((e^{-\gamma})^-)$. Note that $P(x \leq 0) = 0$, as required since $g(x) = -\ln(x)$ is not defined (or at least not real–valued) for $x \leq 0$. We find

$$F_z(\gamma) = \begin{cases} 0, & \gamma < \ln(0.1) \\ 1 - e^{-0.1\gamma}, & \ln(0.1) \leq \gamma. \end{cases}$$ ■

The previous examples illustrated evaluating the probability distribution of a function of a continuous random variable using the CDF technique. This technique is applicable for all functions $z = g(x)$, continuous and discontinuous. Additionally, the CDF technique is applicable if random variable x is mixed or discrete. For mixed random variables, the CDF technique is used without any changes or modifications as shown in the next example.

Example 6.1.6. *Random variable x has PDF*

$$f_x(\alpha) = 0.5(u(\alpha) - u(\alpha-1)) + 0.5\delta(\alpha - 0.5).$$

Find the CDF for $z = g(x) = 1/x^2$.

52 ADVANCED PROBABILITY THEORY FOR BIOMEDICAL ENGINEERS

Solution. The mixed random variable x has CDF

$$F_x(\alpha) = \begin{cases} 0, & \alpha < 0 \\ 0.5\alpha, & 0 \leq \alpha < 0.5 \\ 0.5 + 0.5\alpha, & 0.5 \leq \alpha < 1 \\ 1, & 1 \leq \alpha. \end{cases}$$

For $\gamma < 0$, $F_z(\gamma) = 0$. For $\gamma > 0$,

$$A(\gamma) = \{x : x^{-2} \leq \gamma\} = \left(-\infty, -\frac{1}{\sqrt{\gamma}}\right] \cup \left[\frac{1}{\sqrt{\gamma}}, \infty\right),$$

so that

$$F_z(\gamma) = F_x(-1/\sqrt{\gamma}) + 1 - F_x((1/\sqrt{\gamma})^-).$$

Since $F_x(-1/\sqrt{\gamma}) = 0$ for all real γ, we have

$$F_z(\gamma) = 1 - \begin{cases} 0, & (1/\sqrt{\gamma})^- < 0 \\ 0.5\gamma^{-1/2}, & 0 \leq (1/\sqrt{\gamma})^- < 0.5 \\ 0.5 + 0.5\gamma^{-1/2}, & 0.5 \leq (1/\sqrt{\gamma})^- < 1 \\ 1, & 1 \leq (1/\sqrt{\gamma})^-. \end{cases}$$

After some algebra,

$$F_z(\gamma) = \begin{cases} 0, & \gamma < 1 \\ 0.5 - 0.5\gamma^{-1/2}, & 1 \leq \gamma < 4 \\ 1 - 0.5\gamma^{-1/2}, & 4 \leq \gamma. \end{cases}$$

∎

Drill Problem 6.1.1. *Random variable x is uniformly distributed in the interval -1 to 4. Random variable $z = 3x + 2$. Determine: (a) $F_z(0)$, (b) $F_z(1)$, (c) $f_z(0)$, (c) $f_z(15)$.*

Answers: 0, 2/15, 1/15, 1/15.

Drill Problem 6.1.2. *Random variable x has the PDF*

$$f_x(\alpha) = 0.5\alpha(u(\alpha) - u(\alpha - 2)).$$

Random variable z is defined by

$$z = \begin{cases} -1, & x < 1 \\ x, & -1 \leq x \leq 1 \\ 1, & x > 1. \end{cases}$$

Determine: (a) $F_z(-1/2)$, (b) $F_z(1/2)$, (c) $F_z(3/2)$, (d) $f_z(1/2)$.
Answers: 0, 1, 1/16, 1/4.

Drill Problem 6.1.3. *Random variable x has the PDF*

$$f_x(\alpha) = 0.5\alpha(u(\alpha) - u(\alpha - 2)).$$

Random variable z is defined by

$$z = \begin{cases} -1, & x \leq 0.5 \\ x + 0.5, & 0.5 < x \leq 1 \\ 3, & x > 1. \end{cases}$$

Determine: (a) $F_z(-1)$, (b) $F_z(0)$, (c) $F_z(3/2)$, (d) $F_z(4)$.
Answers: 1/4, 1/16, 1/16, 1.

Drill Problem 6.1.4. *Random variable x has PDF*

$$f_x(\alpha) = e^{-\alpha - 1} u(\alpha + 1).$$

Random variable $z = 1/x^2$. Determine: (a) $F_z(1/8)$, (b) $F_z(1/2)$, (c) $F_z(4)$, (d) $f_z(4)$.

Answers: 0.0519, 0.617, 0.089, 0.022.

6.2 UNIVARIATE PDF TECHNIQUE

The previous section solved the problem of determining the probability distribution of a function of a random variable using the cumulative distribution function. Now, we introduce a second method for calculating the probability distribution of a function $z = g(x)$ using the probability density function, called the PDF technique. The PDF technique, however, is only applicable for functions of random variables in which $z = g(x)$ is continuous and does not equal a constant in any interval in which f_x is nonzero. We introduce the PDF technique for two reasons. First, in many situations it is much simpler to use than the CDF technique. Second, we will find the PDF method most useful in extensions to multivariate functions. In this section, we discuss a wide variety of situations using the PDF technique with functions of continuous random variables. Then, a method for handling mixed random variables with the PDF technique is introduced. Finally, we consider computing the conditional PDF of a function of a random variable using the PDF technique.

6.2.1 Continuous Random Variable

Theorem 6.2.1. *Let x be a continuous RV with PDF $f_x(\alpha)$ and let the RV $z = g(x)$. Assume g is continuous and not constant over any interval for which $f_x \neq 0$. Let*

$$\alpha_i = \alpha_i(\gamma) = g^{-1}(\gamma), \quad i = 1, 2, \ldots, \tag{6.11}$$

denote the distinct solutions to $g(\alpha_i) = \gamma$. Then

$$f_z(\gamma) = \sum_{i=1}^{\infty} \frac{f_x(\alpha_i(\gamma))}{|g^{(1)}(\alpha_i(\gamma))|}, \qquad (6.12)$$

where we interpret

$$\frac{f_x(\alpha_i(\gamma))}{|g^{(1)}(\alpha_i(\gamma))|} = 0,$$

if $f_x(\alpha_i(\gamma)) = 0$.

Proof. Let $h > 0$ and define

$$I(\gamma, h) = \{x : \gamma - h < g(x) \leq \gamma\}.$$

Partition $I(\gamma, h)$ into disjoint intervals of the form

$$I_i(\gamma, h) = (a_i(\gamma, h), b_i(\gamma, h)), \quad i = 1, 2, \ldots,$$

such that

$$I(\gamma, h) = \bigcup_{i=1}^{\infty} I_i(\gamma, h).$$

Then

$$F_z(\gamma) - F_z(\gamma - h) = \sum_{i=1}^{\infty} (F_x(b_i(\gamma, h)) - F_x(a_i(\gamma, h)))$$

By hypothesis,

$$\lim_{h \to 0} a_i(\gamma, h) = \lim_{h \to 0} b_i(\gamma, h) = \alpha_i(\gamma).$$

Note that (for all γ with $f_x(\alpha_i(\gamma)) \neq 0$)

$$\lim_{h \to 0} \frac{b_i(\gamma, h) - a_i(\gamma, h)}{h} = \lim_{h \to 0} \frac{b_i(\gamma, h) - a_i(\gamma, h)}{|g(b_i(\gamma, h)) - g(a_i(\gamma, h))|} = \frac{1}{|g^{(1)}(\alpha_i(\gamma))|},$$

and that

$$\lim_{h \to 0} \frac{F_x(b_i(\gamma, h)) - F_x(a_i(\gamma, h))}{b_i(\gamma, h) - a_i(\gamma, h)} = f_x(\alpha_i(\gamma)).$$

The desired result follows by taking the product of the above limits. The absolute value appears because by construction we have $b_i > a_i$ and $h > 0$, whereas $g^{(1)}$ may be positive or negative. ∎

Example 6.2.1. *Random variable x is uniformly distributed in the interval 0–4. Find the PDF for random variable $z = g(x) = 2x + 1$.*

Solution. In this case, there is only one solution to the equation $\gamma = 2\alpha + 1$, given by $\alpha_1 = (\gamma - 1)/2$. We easily find $g^{(1)}(\alpha) = 2$. Hence

$$f_z(\gamma) = f_x((\gamma - 1)/2)/2 = \begin{cases} 1/8, & 1 < \gamma < 9 \\ 0, & \text{otherwise.} \end{cases}$$

■

Example 6.2.2. *Random variable x has PDF*

$$f_x(\alpha) = 0.75(1 - \alpha^2)(u(\alpha + 1) - u(\alpha - 1)).$$

Find the PDF for random variable $z = g(x) = 1/x^2$.

Solution. For $\gamma < 0$, there are no solutions to $g(\alpha_i) = \gamma$, so that $f_z(\gamma) = 0$ for $\gamma < 0$. For $\gamma > 0$ there are two solutions to $g(\alpha_i) = \gamma$:

$$\alpha_1(\gamma) = -\frac{1}{\sqrt{\gamma}}, \quad \text{and} \quad \alpha_2(\gamma) = \frac{1}{\sqrt{\gamma}}.$$

Since $\gamma = g(\alpha) = \alpha^{-2}$, we have $g^{(1)}(\alpha) = -2\alpha^{-3}$; hence, $|g^{(1)}(\alpha_i)| = 2/|\alpha_i|^3 = 2|\gamma|^{3/2}$, and

$$f_z(\gamma) = \frac{f_x(-\gamma^{-1/2}) + f_x(\gamma^{-1/2})}{2\gamma^{3/2}} u(\gamma).$$

Substituting,

$$f_z(\gamma) = \frac{0.75(1 - \gamma^{-1})(u(1 - \gamma^{-1/2}) - 0 + 1 - u(\gamma^{-1/2} - 1))}{2\gamma^{3/2}} u(\gamma).$$

Simplifying,

$$f_z(\gamma) = \frac{0.75(1 - \gamma^{-1})(u(\gamma - 1) - 0 + 1 - u(1 - \gamma))}{2\gamma^{3/2}} u(\gamma),$$

or

$$f_z(\gamma) = 0.75(\gamma^{-\frac{3}{2}} - \gamma^{-\frac{5}{2}})u(\gamma - 1).$$

■

Example 6.2.3. *Random variable x has PDF*

$$f_x(\alpha) = \frac{1}{6}(1 + \alpha^2)(u(\alpha + 1) - u(\alpha - 2)).$$

Find the PDF for random variable $z = g(x) = x^2$.

Solution. For $\gamma<0$ there are no solutions to $g(\alpha_i)=\gamma$, so that $f_z(\gamma)=0$ for $\gamma<0$. For $\gamma>0$ there are two solutions to $g(\alpha_i)=\gamma$:

$$\alpha_1(\gamma)=-\sqrt{\gamma}, \quad \text{and} \quad \alpha_2(\gamma)=\sqrt{\gamma}.$$

Since $\gamma=g(\alpha)=\alpha^2$, we have $g^{(1)}(\alpha)=2\alpha$; hence, $|g^{(1)}(\alpha_i)|=2|\alpha_i|=2\sqrt{\gamma}$, and

$$f_z(\gamma)=\frac{f_x(-\sqrt{\gamma})+f_x(\sqrt{\gamma})}{2\sqrt{\gamma}}u(\gamma).$$

Substituting,

$$f_z(\gamma)=\frac{1+\gamma}{12\sqrt{\gamma}}(u(1-\sqrt{\gamma})-u(-2-\sqrt{\gamma})+u(\sqrt{\gamma}+1)-u(\sqrt{\gamma}-2))u(\gamma).$$

Simplifying,

$$f_z(\gamma)=\frac{1+\gamma}{12\sqrt{\gamma}}(u(1-\gamma)-0+1-u(\gamma-4))u(\gamma),$$

or

$$f_z(\gamma)=\begin{cases}(\gamma^{-1/2}+\gamma^{1/2})/6, & 0<\gamma<1\\ (\gamma^{-1/2}+\gamma^{1/2})/12, & 1<\gamma<4\\ 0, & \text{elsewhere.}\end{cases}$$

∎

6.2.2 Mixed Random Variable

Consider the problem where random variable x is mixed, and we wish to find the PDF for $z=g(x)$. Here, we treat the discrete and continuous portions of f_x separately, and then combine the results to yield f_z. The continuous part of the PDF of x is handled by the PDF technique. To illustrate the use of this technique, consider the following example.

Example 6.2.4. *Random variable x has PDF*

$$f_x(\alpha)=\frac{3}{8}(u(\alpha+1)-u(\alpha-1))+\frac{1}{8}\delta(\alpha+0.5)+\frac{1}{8}\delta(\alpha-0.5).$$

Find the PDF for the RV $z=g(x)=e^{-x}$.

Solution. There is only one solution to $g(\alpha)=\gamma$:

$$\alpha_1(\gamma)=-\ln(\gamma).$$

We have $g^{(1)}(\alpha_1)=-e^{\ln(\gamma)}=-\gamma$. The probability masses of 1/8 for x at -0.5 and 0.5 are mapped to probability masses of 1/8 for z at $e^{0.5}$ and $e^{-0.5}$, respectively. For all $\gamma>0$ such that

$|\alpha_1(\gamma) \pm 0.5| > 0$ we have
$$f_z(\gamma) = \frac{f_x(-\ln(\gamma))}{\gamma}.$$

Combining these results, we find
$$f_z(\gamma) = \frac{3}{8\gamma}(u(\gamma - e^{-1}) - u(\gamma - e)) + \frac{1}{8}\delta(\gamma - e^{0.5}) + \frac{1}{8}\delta(\gamma - e^{-0.5}).$$ ∎

6.2.3 Conditional PDF Technique

Since a conditional PDF is also a PDF, the above techniques apply to find the conditional PDF for $z = g(x)$, given event A. Consider the problem where random variable x has PDF f_x, and we wish to evaluate the conditional PDF for random variable $z = g(x)$, given that event A occurred. Depending on whether the event A is defined on the range or domain of $z = g(x)$, one of the following two methods may be used to determine the conditional PDF of z using the PDF technique.

(i) If A is an event defined for an interval on z, the conditional PDF, $f_{z|A}$, is computed by first evaluating f_z using the technique in this section. Then, by the definition of a conditional PDF, we have
$$f_{z|A}(\gamma|A) = \frac{f_z(\gamma)}{P(A)}, \qquad \gamma \in A, \qquad (6.13)$$
and $f_{z|A}(\gamma|A) = 0$ for $\gamma \notin A$.

(ii) If A is an event defined for an interval on x, we will use the conditional PDF of x to evaluate the conditional PDF for z as
$$f_{z|A}(\gamma|A) = \sum_{i=1}^{\infty} \frac{f_{x|A}(\alpha_i(\gamma)|A)}{|g^{(1)}(\alpha_i(\gamma))|}. \qquad (6.14)$$

Example 6.2.5. *Random variable x has the PDF*
$$f_x(\alpha) = \frac{1}{6}(1 + \alpha^2)(u(\alpha + 1) - u(\alpha - 2)).$$
Find the PDF for random variable $z = g(x) = x^2$, given $A = \{x : x > 0\}$.

Solution. First, we solve for the conditional PDF for x and then find the conditional PDF for z, based on $f_{x|A}$. We have
$$P(A) = \frac{1}{6}\int_0^2 (1+\alpha^2)d\alpha = \frac{7}{9},$$

so that

$$f_{x|A}(\alpha|A) = \frac{3}{14}(1+\alpha^2)(u(\alpha) - u(\alpha - 2)).$$

There is only one solution to $\gamma = g(\alpha) = \alpha^2$ on the interval $0 < \alpha < 2$ where $f_{x|A} \neq 0$. We have $\alpha_1(\gamma) = \sqrt{\gamma}$ and $|g^{(1)}(\alpha_1(\gamma))| = 2\sqrt{\gamma}$. Consequently,

$$f_{z|A}(\gamma|A) = \frac{3}{28}\left(\sqrt{\gamma} + \frac{1}{\sqrt{\gamma}}\right)(u(\gamma) - u(\gamma - 4)).$$ ∎

Drill Problem 6.2.1. *Random variable x has a uniform PDF in the interval 0–8. Random variable $z = 3x + 1$. Use the PDF method to determine: (a) $f_z(0)$, (b) $f_z(6)$, (c) $E(z)$, (d) σ_z^2.*

Answers: 13, 48, 0, 1/24.

Drill Problem 6.2.2. *Random variable x has the PDF*

$$f_x(\alpha) = \begin{cases} 9\alpha^2, & 0 \leq \alpha < 0.5 \\ 3(1-\alpha^2), & 0.5 \leq \alpha \leq 1 \\ 0, & \text{otherwise.} \end{cases}$$

Random variable $z = x^3$. Use the PDF method to determine: (a) $f_z(1/27)$, (b) $f_z(1/4)$, (c) $f_{z|z>1/8}(1/4|z > 1/8)$, (d) $f_z(2)$.

Answers: 1.52, 0, 3, 2.43.

Drill Problem 6.2.3. *Random variable x has the PDF*

$$f_x(\alpha) = \frac{2}{9}\alpha(u(\alpha) - u(\alpha - 3)).$$

Random variable $z = (x-1)^2$. Use the PDF method to determine: (a) $f_z(1/4)$, (b) $f_z(9/4)$, (c) $f_{z|z\leq 1}(1/4|z \leq 1)$, (d) $E(z|z \leq 1)$.

Answers: 4/9, 5/27, 1/3, 1.

Drill Problem 6.2.4. *Random variable x has the PDF*

$$f_x(\alpha) = \frac{2}{9}(\alpha+1)(u(\alpha+1) - u(\alpha-2)).$$

Random variable $z = 2x^2$ and event $A = \{x : x \geq 0\}$. Determine: (a) $P(A)$, (b) $f_{x|A}(1|A)$, (c) $f_{z|A}(2|A)$, (d) $f_{z|A}(9|A)$.

Answers: 0, 1/2, 1/8, 8/9.

6.3 ONE FUNCTION OF TWO RANDOM VARIABLES

Consider a random variable $z = g(x, y)$ created from jointly distributed random variables x and y. In this section, the probability distribution of $z = g(x, y)$ is computed using a CDF technique similar to the one at the start of this chapter. Because we are dealing with regions in a plane instead of intervals on a line, these problems are not as straightforward and tractable as before.

With $z = g(x, y)$, we have

$$F_z(\gamma) = P(z \le \gamma) = P(g(x, y) \le \gamma) = P((x, y) \in A(\gamma)), \quad (6.15)$$

where

$$A(\gamma) = \{(x, y) : g(x, y) \le \gamma\}. \quad (6.16)$$

The CDF for the RV z can then be found by evaluating the integral

$$F_z(\gamma) = \int_{A(\gamma)} dF_{x,y}(\alpha, \beta). \quad (6.17)$$

This result cannot be continued further until a specific $F_{x,y}$ and $g(x, y)$ are considered. Remember that in the case of a single random variable, our efforts primarily dealt with algebraic manipulations. Here, our efforts are concentrated on evaluating F_z through integrals, with the ease of solution critically dependent on $g(x, y)$.

The ease in solution for F_z is dependent on transforming $A(\gamma)$ into proper limits of integration. Sketching the support region for $f_{x,y}$ (the region where $f_{x,y} \ne 0$, or $F_{x,y}$ is not constant) and the region $A(\gamma)$ is often most helpful, even crucial, in the problem solution. Pay careful attention to the limits of integration to determine the range of integration in which the integrand is zero because $f_{x,y} = 0$. Let us consider several examples to illustrate the mechanics of the CDF technique and also to provide further insight.

Example 6.3.1. *Random variables x and y have joint PDF*

$$f_{x,y}(\alpha, \beta) = \begin{cases} 1/4, & 0 < \alpha < 2, 0 < \beta < 2 \\ 0, & \text{otherwise.} \end{cases}$$

Find the CDF for $z = x + y$.

Solution. We have $A(\gamma) = \{(\alpha, \beta) : \alpha + \beta \le \gamma\}$. We require the volume under the surface $f_{x,y}(\alpha, \beta)$ where $\alpha \le \gamma - \beta$:

$$F_z(\gamma) = \int_{-\infty}^{\infty} \int_{-\infty}^{\gamma-\beta} f_{x,y}(\alpha, \beta) d\alpha \, d\beta.$$

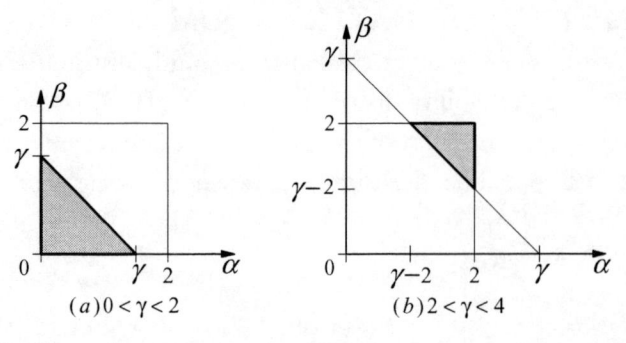

60 ADVANCED PROBABILITY THEORY FOR BIOMEDICAL ENGINEERS

FIGURE 6.3: Plots for Example 6.3.1.

For $\gamma < 0$ we have $F_z(\gamma) = 0$. For $0 \le \gamma < 2$, with the aid of Figure 6.3(a) we obtain

$$F_z(\gamma) = \int_0^2 \int_0^{\gamma-\beta} \frac{1}{4} d\alpha\, d\beta = \frac{1}{8}\gamma^2.$$

For $2 \le \gamma < 4$, referring to Figure 6.3(b), we consider the complementary region (to save some work):

$$F_z(\gamma) = 1 - \int_{\gamma-2}^2 \int_{\gamma-\beta}^2 \frac{1}{4} d\alpha\, d\beta = 1 - \frac{1}{8}(4 - \gamma)^2.$$

Finally, for $4 \le \gamma$, $F_z(\gamma) = 1$. ∎

Example 6.3.2. *Random variables x and y have joint PDF*

$$f_{x,y}(\alpha, \beta) = \begin{cases} 1, & 0 < \alpha < 1, 0 < \beta < 1 \\ 0, & \text{otherwise.} \end{cases}$$

Find the PDF for $z = x - y$.

Solution. We have $A(\gamma) = \{(\alpha, \beta) : \alpha - \beta \le \gamma\}$. We require the volume under the surface $f_{x,y}(\alpha, \beta)$ where $\alpha \le \gamma + \beta$:

$$F_z(\gamma) = \int_{-\infty}^{\infty} \int_{-\infty}^{\gamma+\beta} f_{x,y}(\alpha, \beta) d\alpha\, d\beta.$$

For $\gamma < -1$ we have $F_z(\gamma) = 0$ and $f_z(\gamma) = 0$. With the aid of Figure 6.4(a), for $-1 \le \gamma < 0$,

$$F_z(\gamma) = \int_{-\gamma}^1 \int_0^{\gamma+\beta} d\alpha\, d\beta = \frac{1}{2}(1 + \gamma)^2,$$

TRANSFORMATIONS OF RANDOM VARIABLES   61

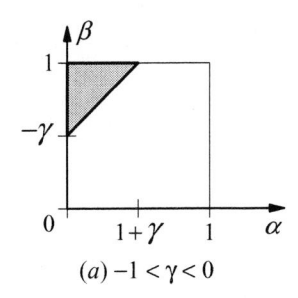

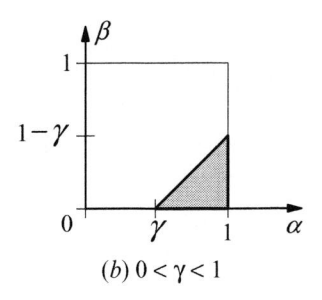

FIGURE 6.4: Plots for Example 6.3.2.

so that $f_z(\gamma) = 1 + \gamma$. For $0 \leq \gamma < 1$, we consider the complementary region shown in Figure 6.4(b) (to save some work):

$$F_z(\gamma) = 1 - \int_0^{1-\gamma} \int_{\gamma+\beta}^1 d\alpha\, d\beta = 1 - \frac{1}{2}(1-\gamma)^2,$$

so that $f_z(\gamma) = 1 - \gamma$. Finally, for $1 \leq \gamma$, $F_z(\gamma) = 1$, so that $f_z(\gamma) = 0$. ∎

Example 6.3.3. *Find the CDF for $z = x/y$, where x and y have the joint PDF*

$$f_{x,y}(\alpha, \beta) = \begin{cases} 1/\alpha, & 0 < \beta < \alpha < 1 \\ 0, & \text{otherwise.} \end{cases}$$

Solution. We have $A(\gamma) = \{(\alpha, \beta) : \alpha/\beta \leq \gamma\}$. Inside the support region for $f_{x,y}$, we have $\alpha/\beta > 1$; hence, for $\gamma < 1$ we have $F_z(\gamma) = 0$. As shown in Figure 6.5 it is easiest to integrate with respect to β first: for $1 \leq \gamma$,

$$F_z(\gamma) = \int_0^1 \int_{\alpha/\gamma}^\alpha \frac{1}{\alpha} d\beta\, d\alpha = 1 - \frac{1}{\gamma}.$$ ∎

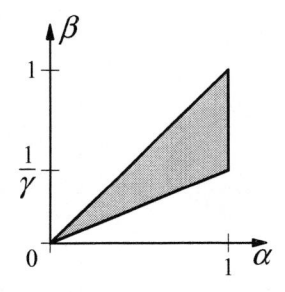

FIGURE 6.5: Integration region for Example 6.3.3.

Example 6.3.4. *Find the CDF for $z = x^2 + y^2$, where x and y have the joint PDF*

$$f_{x,y}(\alpha, \beta) = \begin{cases} 3\alpha, & 0 < \beta < \alpha < 1 \\ 0, & \text{otherwise.} \end{cases}$$

Solution. We have $A(\gamma) = \{(\alpha, \beta) : \alpha^2 + \beta^2 \leq \gamma\}$. For $\gamma < 0$, we obtain $F_z(\gamma) = 0$. Transforming to polar coordinates: $\alpha = r\cos(\theta)$, $\beta = r\sin(\theta)$,

$$F_z(\gamma) = \int_0^{2\pi} \int_{r^2 \leq \gamma} f_{x,y}(r\cos(\theta), r\sin(\theta)) r\, dr\, d\theta.$$

Referring to Figure 6.6(a), for $0 \leq \gamma < 1$,

$$F_z(\gamma) = \int_0^{\pi/4} \int_0^{\sqrt{\gamma}} 3r^2 \cos(\theta) dr\, d\theta = \frac{1}{\sqrt{2}} \gamma^{\frac{3}{2}}.$$

For $1 \leq \gamma < 2$, we split the integral into two parts: one with polar coordinates, the other using rectangular coordinates. With

$$\sin(\theta_1) = \frac{\sqrt{\gamma - 1}}{\sqrt{\gamma}},$$

we find with the aid of Figure 6.6(b) that

$$F_z(\gamma) = \int_{\theta_1}^{\pi/4} \int_0^{\sqrt{\gamma}} 3r^2 \cos(\theta) dr\, d\theta + \int_0^1 \int_0^{\alpha\sqrt{\gamma-1}} 3\alpha\, d\beta\, d\alpha,$$

or

$$F_z(\gamma) = \frac{1}{\sqrt{2}} \gamma^{\frac{3}{2}} - (\gamma - 1)^{\frac{3}{2}}.$$

Finally, we have $F_z(\gamma) = 1$ for $2 \leq \gamma$. ∎

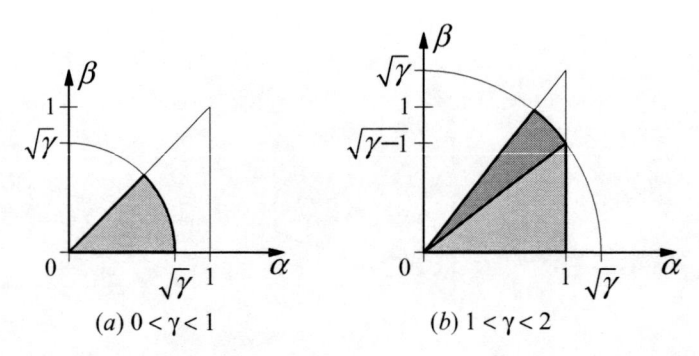

FIGURE 6.6: Integration regions for Example 6.3.4.

Drill Problem 6.3.1. *Random variables x and y have joint PDF*

$$f_{x,y}(\alpha, \beta) = e^{-\alpha} e^{-\beta} u(\alpha) u(\beta).$$

Random variable $z = x - y$. Find (a) $F_z(-1/3)$, (b) $f_z(-1)$, (c) $F_z(1)$, and (d) $f_z(1)$.

Answers: $\frac{1}{4}e^{-1}$, $\frac{3}{4}e^{-1}$, $1 - \frac{3}{4}e^{-1}$, $\frac{3}{4}e^{-1}$.

6.4 BIVARIATE TRANSFORMATIONS

In this section, we find the joint distribution of random variables $z = g(x, y)$ and $w = h(x, y)$ from jointly distributed random variables x and y. First, we consider a bivariate CDF technique. Then, the joint PDF technique for finding the joint PDF for random variables z and w formed from x and y is described. Next, the case of one function of two random variables is treated by using the joint PDF technique with an auxiliary random variable. Finally, the conditional joint PDF is presented.

6.4.1 Bivariate CDF Technique

Let x and y be jointly distributed RVs on the probability space $(S, \Im, P)$, and let $z = g(x, y)$ and $w = h(x, y)$. Define $A(\gamma, \psi)$ to be the region of the $x - y$ plane for which $z = g(x, y) \leq \gamma$ and $w = h(x, y) \leq \psi$; i.e.,

$$A(\gamma, \psi) = \{(x, y) : g(x, y) \leq \gamma, h(x, y) \leq \psi\}. \tag{6.18}$$

Note that

$$A(\gamma, \psi) = g^{-1}((-\infty, \gamma]) \cap h^{-1}((-\infty, \psi]). \tag{6.19}$$

Then

$$F_{z,w}(\gamma, \psi) = \int_{A(\gamma,\psi)} \int dF_{x,y}(\alpha, \beta). \tag{6.20}$$

It is often difficult to perform the integration indicated in (6.20).

Example 6.4.1. *Random variables x and y have the joint PDF*

$$f_{x,y}(\alpha, \beta) = \begin{cases} 0.25, & 0 \leq \alpha \leq 2, 0 \leq \beta \leq 2 \\ 0, & \text{otherwise.} \end{cases}$$

With $z = g(x, y) = x + y$ and $w = h(x, y) = y$, find the joint PDF $f_{z,w}$.

Solution. We have

$$g^{-1}((-\infty, \gamma]) = \{(x, y) : x + y \leq \gamma\}$$

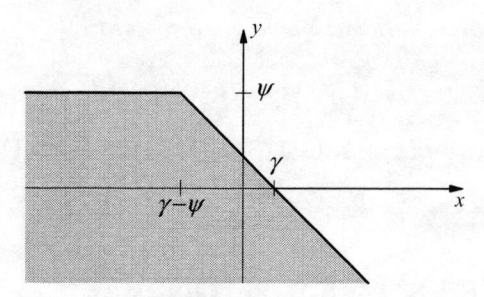

FIGURE 6.7: Integration region for Example 6.4.1.

and
$$h^{-1}((-\infty, \psi]) = \{(x, y) : y \leq \psi\}.$$

The intersection of these regions is
$$A(\gamma, \psi) = \{(x, y) : y \leq \min(\gamma - x, \psi)\},$$

which is illustrated in Figure. 6.7. With the aid of Figure 6.7 and (6.20) we find
$$F_{z,w}(\gamma, \psi) = \int_{-\infty}^{\psi} \int_{-\infty}^{\gamma-\beta} dF_{x,y}(\alpha, \beta).$$

Instead of carrying out the above integration and then differentiating the result, we differentiate the above integral to obtain the PDF $f_{z,w}$ directly. We find
$$\frac{\partial F_{z,w}(\gamma, \psi)}{\partial \gamma} = \lim_{h_1 \to 0} \frac{1}{h_1} \int_{-\infty}^{\psi} \int_{\gamma-h_1-\beta}^{\gamma-\beta} dF_{x,y}(\alpha, \beta),$$

and
$$\frac{\partial^2 F_{z,w}(\gamma, \psi)}{\partial \psi \, \partial \gamma} = \lim_{h_2 \to 0} \lim_{h_1 \to 0} \frac{1}{h_1 h_2} \int_{\psi-h_2}^{\psi} \int_{\gamma-h_1-\beta}^{\gamma-\beta} dF_{x,y}(\alpha, \beta).$$

Performing the indicated limits, we find that $f_{z,w}(\gamma, \psi) = f_{x,y}(\gamma - \psi, \psi)$; substituting, we obtain
$$f_{z,w}(\gamma, \psi) = \begin{cases} 0.25, & 0 < \gamma - \psi < 2, 0 < \psi < 2 \\ 0, & \text{otherwise.} \end{cases}$$ ∎

When the RVs x and y are jointly continuous, it is usually easier to find the joint PDF $f_{z,w}$ than to carry out the integral indicated in (6.20).

6.4.2 Bivariate PDF Technique

A very important special case of bivariate transformations is when the RVs x and y are jointly continuous RVs and the mapping determined by g and h is continuous with g and h having continuous partial derivatives. Let $h_1 > 0$, $h_2 > 0$ and define

$$I(\gamma, h_1, \psi, h_2) = g^{-1}((\gamma - h_1, \gamma]) \cap h^{-1}((\psi - h_2, \psi]). \qquad (6.21)$$

Partition I into disjoint regions so that

$$I(\gamma, h_1, \psi, h_2) = \bigcup_i I_i(\gamma, h_1, \psi, h_2). \qquad (6.22)$$

Let (α_i, β_i) denote the unique element of

$$\lim_{h_1 \to 0} \lim_{h_2 \to 0} I_i(\gamma, h_1, \psi, h_2).$$

Then for small h_1 and small h_2 we have

$$h_1 h_2 f_{v,w}(\gamma, \psi) \approx \sum_i f_{x,y}(\alpha_i, \beta_i) \int_{I_i(\gamma, h_1, \psi, h_2)} d\alpha \, d\beta. \qquad (6.23)$$

Dividing both sides of the above by $h_1 h_2$ and letting $h_1 \to 0$ and $h_2 \to 0$, the approximation becomes an equality. The result is summarized by the theorem below.

Theorem 6.4.1. *Let x and y be jointly continuous RVs with PDF $f_{x,y}$, and let $z = g(x, y)$ and $w = h(x, y)$. Let*

$$(\alpha_i(\gamma, \psi), \beta_i(\gamma, \psi)), \quad i = 1, 2, \ldots, \qquad (6.24)$$

be the distinct solutions to the simultaneous equations

$$g(\alpha_i, \beta_i) = \gamma \qquad (6.25)$$

and

$$h(\alpha_i, \beta_i) = \psi. \qquad (6.26)$$

Define the Jacobian

$$J(\alpha, \beta) = \begin{vmatrix} \dfrac{\partial g(\alpha, \beta)}{\partial \alpha} & \dfrac{\partial g(\alpha, \beta)}{\partial \beta} \\ \dfrac{\partial h(\alpha, \beta)}{\partial \alpha} & \dfrac{\partial h(\alpha, \beta)}{\partial \beta} \end{vmatrix}, \qquad (6.27)$$

where the indicated partial derivatives are assumed to exist. Then

$$f_{z,w}(\gamma, \psi) = \sum_{i=1}^{\infty} \frac{f_{x,y}(\alpha_i, \beta_i)}{|J(\alpha_i, \beta_i)|}. \tag{6.28}$$

The most difficult aspects to finding $f_{z,w}$ using the joint PDF technique are solving the simultaneous equations $\gamma = g(\alpha_i, \beta_i)$ and $\psi = h(\alpha_i, \beta_i)$ for α_i and β_i, and determining the support region for $f_{z,w}$. Let us consider several examples to illustrate the mechanics of this PDF technique.

Example 6.4.2. *Random variables x and y have the joint PDF*

$$f_{x,y}(\alpha, \beta) = \begin{cases} 1/4, & 0 < \alpha < 2, 0 < \beta < 2 \\ 0, & \text{otherwise.} \end{cases}$$

Find the joint PDF for $z = g(x, y) = x + y$ *and* $w = h(x, y) = y$.

Solution. There is only one solution to $\gamma = \alpha + \beta$ and $\psi = \beta$: $\alpha_1 = \gamma - \psi$ and $\beta_1 = \psi$. The Jacobian of the transformation is

$$J = \begin{vmatrix} 1 & 1 \\ 0 & 1 \end{vmatrix} = 1 \cdot 1 - 1 \cdot 0 = 1.$$

Applying Theorem 1, we find

$$f_{z,w}(\gamma, \psi) = \frac{f_{x,y}(\alpha_1, \beta_1)}{|J|} = f_{x,y}(\gamma - \psi, \psi).$$

Substituting, we obtain

$$f_{z,w}(\gamma, \psi) = \begin{cases} 1/4, & 0 < \gamma - \psi < 2, 0 < \psi < 2 \\ 0, & \text{otherwise.} \end{cases}$$

The region of support for $f_{z,w}$ is illustrated in Figure 6.8. ∎

Example 6.4.3. *Random variables x and y have the joint PDF*

$$f_{x,y}(\alpha, \beta) = \begin{cases} 12\alpha\beta(1 - \alpha), & 0 < \alpha < 1, 0 < \beta < 1 \\ 0, & \text{otherwise.} \end{cases}$$

Find the joint PDF for $z = g(x, y) = x^2 y$ *and* $w = h(x, y) = y$.

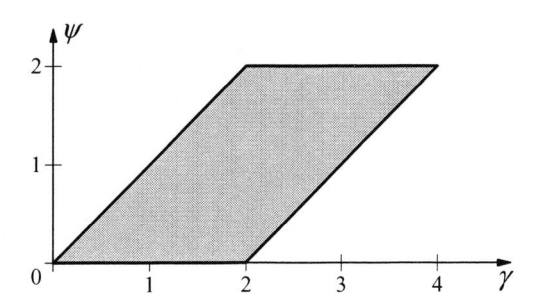

FIGURE 6.8: Support region for Example 6.4.2.

Solution. Solving $\gamma = \alpha^2 \beta$ and $\psi = \beta$, we find $\alpha_1 = \sqrt{\gamma/\psi}$ and $\beta_1 = \psi$. The other solution $\alpha_2 = -\alpha_1$ is not needed since $f_{x,y}(\alpha, \beta) = 0$ for $\alpha < 0$. The Jacobian is

$$J_1 = \begin{vmatrix} 2\alpha_1\beta_1 & \alpha_1^2 \\ 0 & 1 \end{vmatrix} = 2\alpha_1\beta_1 = 2\sqrt{\gamma\psi}.$$

Applying Theorem 1, we find

$$f_{z,w}(\gamma, \psi) = \frac{f_{x,y}(\sqrt{\gamma/\psi}, \psi)}{2\sqrt{\gamma\psi}}$$

$$= \begin{cases} 6(1 - \sqrt{\gamma/\psi}), & 0 < \sqrt{\gamma/\psi} < 1, 0 < \psi < 1 \\ 0, & \text{otherwise.} \end{cases}$$ ∎

Example 6.4.4. *Random variables x and y have the joint PDF*

$$f_{x,y}(\alpha, \beta) = \begin{cases} 0.25(\alpha + 1), & -1 < \alpha < 1, -1 < \beta < 1 \\ 0, & \text{otherwise.} \end{cases}$$

Find the joint PDF for $z = g(x, y) = xy$ and $w = h(x, y) = y/x$.

Solution. Solving $\gamma = \alpha\beta$ and $\psi = \beta/\alpha$, we find $\alpha = \gamma/\beta = \beta/\psi$, so that $\beta^2 = \gamma\psi$. Letting $\beta_1 = \sqrt{\gamma\psi}$ we have $\alpha_1 = \sqrt{\gamma/\psi}$. Then $\beta_2 = -\sqrt{\gamma\psi}$ and $\alpha_2 = -\sqrt{\gamma/\psi}$. Note that the solution (α_1, β_1) is in the first quadrant of the $\alpha - \beta$ plane; the solution (α_2, β_2) is in the third quadrant of the $\alpha - \beta$ plane. We find

$$J = \begin{vmatrix} \beta & \alpha \\ -\beta/\alpha^2 & 1/\alpha \end{vmatrix} = 2\frac{\beta}{\alpha},$$

so that $J_1 = 2\psi = J_2$. Hence

$$f_{z,w}(\gamma, \psi) = \frac{f_{x,y}(\sqrt{\gamma/\psi}, \sqrt{\gamma\psi})}{2|\psi|} + \frac{f_{x,y}(-\sqrt{\gamma/\psi}, -\sqrt{\gamma\psi})}{2|\psi|}.$$

In the $\gamma-\psi$ plane,
$$\frac{f_{x,y}(\sqrt{\gamma/\psi},\sqrt{\gamma\psi})}{2|\psi|}$$
has support region specified by
$$0<\sqrt{\gamma/\psi}<1 \quad \text{and} \quad 0<\sqrt{\gamma\psi}<1,$$
or
$$0<\frac{\gamma}{\psi}<1 \quad \text{and} \quad 0<\gamma\psi<1.$$

Similarly,
$$\frac{f_{x,y}(-\sqrt{\gamma/\psi},-\sqrt{\gamma\psi})}{2|\psi|}$$
has support region specified by
$$-1<-\sqrt{\gamma/\psi}<0 \quad \text{and} \quad -1<-\sqrt{\gamma\psi}<0,$$
or
$$0<\frac{\gamma}{\psi}<1 \quad \text{and} \quad 0<\gamma\psi<1.$$

Consequently, the two components of the PDF $f_{z,w}$ have identical regions of support in the $\gamma-\psi$ plane. In the first quadrant of the $\gamma-\psi$ plane, this support region is easily seen to be $0<\gamma<\psi<\gamma^{-1}$. Similarly, in the third quadrant, the support region is $\gamma^{-1}<\psi<\gamma<0$. This support region is illustrated in Figure 6.9. Finally, we find

$$f_{z,w}(\gamma,\psi) = \begin{cases} 1/(4|\psi|), & 0<\gamma<\psi<\gamma^{-1}, \text{ or } \gamma^{-1}<\psi<\gamma<0 \\ 0, & \text{otherwise.} \end{cases}$$ ∎

Auxiliary Random Variables

The joint PDF technique can also be used to transform random variables x and y with joint PDF $f_{x,y}$ to random variable $z=g(x,y)$ by introducing auxiliary random variable $w=h(x,y)$ to find $f_{z,w}$ and then finding the marginal PDF f_z using

$$f_z(\gamma) = \int_{-\infty}^{\infty} f_{z,w}(\gamma,\psi)d\psi. \tag{6.29}$$

It is usually advisable to let the auxiliary random variable w equal a quantity which allows a convenient solution of the Jacobian and/or the inverse equations. This method is an alternative to the CDF technique presented earlier.

TRANSFORMATIONS OF RANDOM VARIABLES

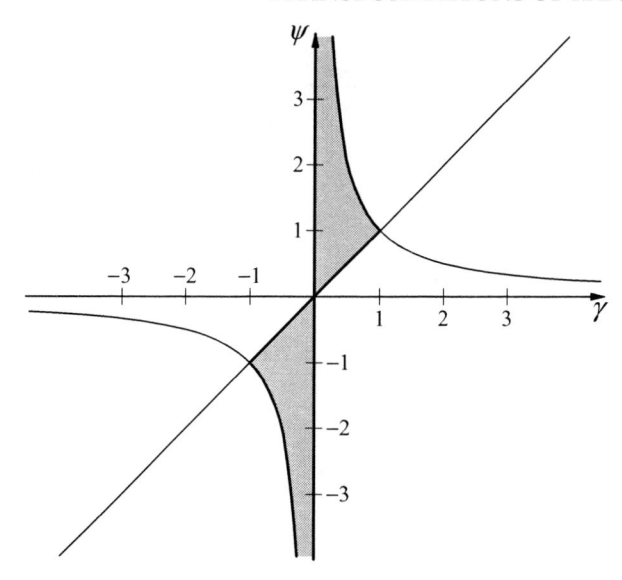

FIGURE 6.9: Support region for Example 6.4.4.

Example 6.4.5. *Random variables x and y have the joint PDF*

$$f_{x,y}(\alpha, \beta) = \begin{cases} 4\alpha\beta, & 0 < \alpha < 1, 0 < \beta < 1 \\ 0, & \text{otherwise.} \end{cases}$$

Find the PDF for $z = g(x, y) = x^2$.

Solution. Let auxiliary variable $w = h(x, y) = y$. Solving $\gamma = \alpha^2$ and $\psi = \beta$, we find $\alpha = \pm\sqrt{\gamma}$ and $\beta = \psi$. The only solution inside the support region for $f_{x,y}$ is $\alpha = \sqrt{\gamma}$ and $\beta = \psi$. The Jacobian of the transformation is

$$J = \begin{vmatrix} 2\alpha & 0 \\ 0 & 1 \end{vmatrix} = 2\alpha,$$

so that

$$f_{z,w}(\gamma, \psi) = \frac{f_{x,y}(\sqrt{\gamma}, \psi)}{2\sqrt{\gamma}} = \begin{cases} \dfrac{4\sqrt{\gamma}\psi}{2\sqrt{\gamma}} = 2\psi, & 0 < \gamma < 1, 0 < \psi < 1 \\ 0, & \text{otherwise.} \end{cases}$$

We find the marginal PDF for z as

$$f_z(\gamma) = \int_{-\infty}^{\infty} f_{z,w}(\gamma, \psi)d\psi = \int_0^1 2\psi\, d\psi.$$

for $0 < \gamma < 1$ and $f_z(\gamma) = 0$, otherwise. ∎

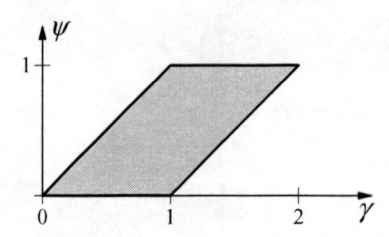

FIGURE 6.10: Support region for Example 6.4.6.

Example 6.4.6. *Random variables x and y have the joint PDF*

$$f_{x,y}(\alpha, \beta) = \begin{cases} 4\alpha\beta, & 0 < \alpha < 1, 0 < \beta < 1 \\ 0, & \text{otherwise.} \end{cases}$$

Find the PDF for $z = g(x, y) = x + y$.

Solution. Let auxiliary variable $w = h(x, y) = y$. Solving $\gamma = \alpha + \beta$ and $\psi = \beta$, we find $\alpha = \gamma - \psi$ and $\beta = \psi$. We find

$$J = \begin{vmatrix} 1 & 1 \\ 0 & 1 \end{vmatrix} = 1,$$

so that

$$f_{z,w}(\gamma, \psi) = f_{x,y}(\gamma - \psi, \psi) = \begin{cases} 4(\gamma - \psi)\psi, & 0 < \gamma - \psi < 1, 0 < \psi < 1 \\ 0, & \text{otherwise.} \end{cases}$$

The support region for $f_{z,w}$ is shown in Figure 6.10. Referring to Figure 6.10, for $0 < \gamma < 1$,

$$f_z(\gamma) = \int_0^\gamma 4(\gamma - \psi)\psi \, d\psi = \frac{2}{3}\gamma^3.$$

For $1 < \gamma < 2$,

$$f_z(\gamma) = \int_{\gamma-1}^1 4(\gamma - \psi)\psi \, d\psi = -\frac{2}{3}\gamma^3 + 4\gamma - \frac{8}{3}.$$

Otherwise, $f_z = 0$. ∎

Conditional PDF Technique
Since a conditional PDF is also a PDF, the above techniques apply to find the conditional PDF for $z = g(x, y)$, given event A. Consider the problem where random variables x and y have joint

TRANSFORMATIONS OF RANDOM VARIABLES 71

PDF $f_{x,y}$, and we wish to evaluate the conditional PDF for random variable $z = g(x, y)$, given that event A occurred. Depending on whether the event A is defined on the range or domain of $z = g(x, y)$, one of the following two methods may be used to determine the conditional PDF of z using the bivariate PDF technique.

i. If A is an event defined for an interval on z, the conditional PDF, $f_{z|A}$, is computed by first evaluating f_z using the technique in this section. Then, by the definition of a conditional PDF, we have

$$f_{z|A}(\gamma|A) = \frac{f_z(\gamma)}{P(A)}, \qquad \gamma \in A. \tag{6.30}$$

ii. If A is an event defined for a region in the $x - y$ plane, we will use the conditional PDF $f_{x,y|A}$ to evaluate the conditional PDF $f_{z|A}$ as follows. First, introduce an auxiliary random variable $w = h(x, y)$, and evaluate

$$f_{z,w|A}(\gamma, \psi|A) = \sum_{i=1}^{\infty} \frac{f_{x,y|A}(\alpha_i(\gamma, \psi), \beta_i(\gamma, \psi)|A)}{|J(\alpha_i(\gamma, \psi), \beta_i(\gamma, \psi))|}, \tag{6.31}$$

where (α_i, β_i), $i = 1, 2, \ldots$, are the solutions to $\gamma = g(\alpha, \beta)$ and $\psi = h(\alpha, \beta)$ in region A. Then evaluate the marginal conditional PDF

$$f_{z|A}(\gamma|A) = \int_{-\infty}^{\infty} f_{z,w|A}(\gamma, \psi|A) d\psi. \tag{6.32}$$

Example 6.4.7. *Random variables x and y have joint PDF*

$$f_{x,y}(\alpha, \beta) = \begin{cases} 3\alpha, & 0 < \beta < \alpha < 1 \\ 0, & \text{otherwise.} \end{cases}$$

Find the PDF for $z = x + y$, given event $A = \{\max(x, y) \leq 0.5\}$.

Solution. We begin by finding the conditional PDF for x and y, given A. From Figure 6.11(a) we find

$$P(A) = \int\!\!\int_A f_{x,y}(\alpha, \beta) d\alpha\, d\beta = \int_0^{0.5} \int_0^{\alpha} 3\alpha\, d\beta\, d\alpha = \frac{1}{8};$$

consequently,

$$f_{x,y|A}(\alpha, \beta|A) = \begin{cases} \dfrac{f_{x,y}(\alpha, \beta)}{P(A)} = 24\alpha, & 0 < \beta < \alpha < 0.5 \\ 0, & \text{otherwise.} \end{cases}$$

72   ADVANCED PROBABILITY THEORY FOR BIOMEDICAL ENGINEERS

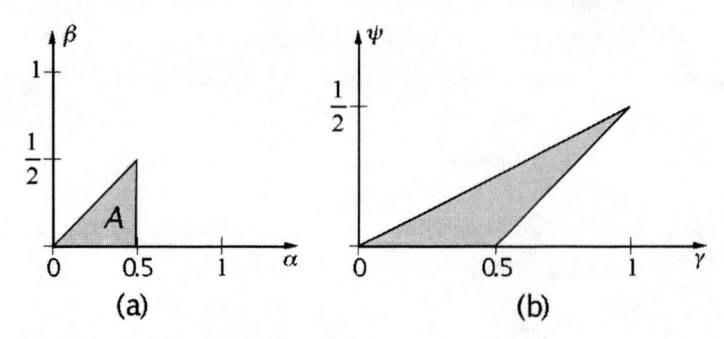

FIGURE 6.11: Support region for Example 6.4.7.

Letting the auxiliary random variable $w = h(x, y) = y$, the only solution to $\gamma = g(\alpha, \beta) = \alpha + \beta$ and $\psi = h(\alpha, \beta) = \beta$ is $\alpha = \gamma - \psi$ and $\beta = \psi$. The Jacobian of the transformation is $J = 1$ so that

$$f_{z,w|A}(\gamma, \psi | A) = \frac{f_{x,y|A}(\gamma - \psi, \psi | A)}{1}.$$

Substituting, we find

$$f_{z,w|A}(\gamma, \psi | A) = \begin{cases} 24(\gamma - \psi), & 0 < \psi < \gamma - \psi < 0.5 \\ 0, & \text{otherwise.} \end{cases}$$

The support region for $f_{z,w|A}$ is illustrated in Figure 6.11(b). The conditional PDF for z, given A, can be found from

$$f_{z|A}(\gamma | A) = \int_{-\infty}^{\infty} f_{z,w|A}(\gamma, \psi | A) d\psi.$$

The integration is easily carried out with the aid of Figure 6.11(b). For $0.5 < \gamma < 1$ we have

$$f_{z|A}(\gamma | A) = \int_{0}^{0.5\gamma} 24(\gamma - \psi) d\psi = 9\gamma^2.$$

For $0.5 < \gamma < 1$ we obtain

$$f_{z|A}(\gamma | A) = \int_{\gamma - 0.5}^{0.5\gamma} 24(\gamma - \psi) d\psi = 3(1 - \gamma^2).$$

For $\gamma < 0$ or $\gamma > 1$, $f_{z|A}(\gamma | A) = 0$. ∎

TRANSFORMATIONS OF RANDOM VARIABLES

Drill Problem 6.4.1. *Random variables x and y have joint PDF*

$$f_{x,y}(\alpha, \beta) = e^{-\alpha-\beta} u(\alpha)u(\beta).$$

Random variable $z = x$ and $w = xy$. Find: (a) $f_{z,w}(1, 1)$, (b) $f_{z,w}(-1, 1)$.

Answers: 0, e^{-2}.

Drill Problem 6.4.2. *Random variables x and y have joint PDF*

$$f_{x,y}(\alpha, \beta) = \begin{cases} 4\alpha\beta, & 0 < \alpha < 1, 0 < \beta < 1 \\ 0, & \text{otherwise.} \end{cases}$$

Random variable $z = x + y$ and $w = y^2$. Determine: (a) $f_{z,w}(1, 1/4)$, (b) $f_z(-1/2)$, (c) $f_z(1/2)$, (d) $f_z(3/2)$.

Answers: 0, 1/12, 1, 13/12.

Drill Problem 6.4.3. *Random variables x and y have joint PDF*

$$f_{x,y}(\alpha, \beta) = \begin{cases} 1.2(\alpha^2 + \beta), & 0 < \alpha < 1, 0 < \beta < 1 \\ 0, & \text{otherwise.} \end{cases}$$

Random variable $z = x^2 y$. Determine: (a) $f_z(-1)$, (b) $f_z(1/4)$, (c) $f_z(1/2)$, (d) $f_z(3/2)$.

Answers: 0.7172, 0, 0, 1.3.

Drill Problem 6.4.4. *Random variables x and y have joint PDF*

$$f_{x,y}(\alpha, \beta) = \begin{cases} 2\beta, & 0 < \alpha < 1, 0 < \beta < 1 \\ 0, & \text{otherwise.} \end{cases}$$

Random variable $z = x - y$ and event $A = \{(x, y) : x + y \leq 1\}$. Determine: (a) $f_{z|A}(-3/2|A)$, (b) $f_{z|A}(-1/2|A)$, (c) $F_{z|A}(0|A)$, (d) $f_{z|A}(1/2|A)$.

Answers: 0, 3/4, 15/16, 3/16.

6.5 SUMMARY

This chapter presented a number of different approaches to find the probability distribution of functions of random variables.

Two methods are presented to find the probability distribution of a function of one random variable, $z = g(x)$. The first, and the most general approach, is called the CDF technique. From the definition of the CDF, we write

$$F_z(\gamma) = P(z \leq \gamma) = P(g(x) \leq \gamma) = P(x \in A(\gamma)), \tag{6.33}$$

where $A(\gamma) = \{x : g(x) \leq \gamma\}$. By partitioning $A(\gamma)$ into disjoint intervals, the CDF F_z may be found using the CDF F_x. The second approach, called the PDF technique, involves evaluating

$$f_z(\gamma) = \sum_{i=1}^{\infty} \frac{f_x(\alpha_i(\gamma))}{|g^{(1)}(\alpha_i(\gamma))|}, \qquad (6.34)$$

where

$$\alpha_i = \alpha_i(\gamma) = g^{-1}(\gamma), \quad i = 1, 2, \ldots, \qquad (6.35)$$

denote the distinct solutions to $g(\alpha_i) = \gamma$. Typically, the PDF technique is much simpler to use than the CDF technique. However, the PDF technique is applicable only when $z = g(x)$ is continuous and does not equal a constant in any interval in which f_x is nonzero.

Next, we evaluated the probability distribution of a random variable $z = g(x, y)$ created from jointly distributed random variables x and y using two approaches. The first approach, a CDF technique, involves evaluating

$$F_z(\gamma) = P(z \leq \gamma) = P(g(x, y) \leq \gamma) = P((x, y) \in A(\gamma)), \qquad (6.36)$$

where

$$A(\gamma) = \{(x, y) : g(x, y) \leq \gamma\}. \qquad (6.37)$$

The CDF for the RV z can then be found by evaluating the integral

$$F_z(\gamma) = \int_{A(\gamma)} dF_{x,y}(\alpha, \beta). \qquad (6.38)$$

The ease of solution here involves transforming $A(\gamma)$ into proper limits of integration. We wish to remind the reader that the special case of a convolution integral is obtained when random variables x and y are independent and $z = x + y$. The second approach involves introducing an auxiliary random variable and using the PDF technique applied to two functions of two random variables.

To find the joint probability distribution of random variables $z = g(x, y)$ and $w = h(x, y)$ from jointly distributed random variables x and y, a bivariate CDF as well as a joint PDF technique were presented. Using the joint PDF technique, the joint PDF for z and w can be found as

$$f_{z,w}(\gamma, \psi) = \sum_{i=1}^{\infty} \frac{f_{x,y}(\alpha_i, \beta_i)}{|J(\alpha_i, \beta_i)|}, \qquad (6.39)$$

where

$$(\alpha_i(\gamma, \psi), \beta_i(\gamma, \psi)), \quad i = 1, 2, \ldots, \qquad (6.40)$$

are the distinct solutions to the simultaneous equations

$$g(\alpha_i, \beta_i) = \gamma \qquad (6.41)$$

and

$$h(\alpha_i, \beta_i) = \psi. \qquad (6.42)$$

The Jacobian

$$J(\alpha, \beta) = \begin{vmatrix} \dfrac{\partial g(\alpha, \beta)}{\partial \alpha} & \dfrac{\partial g(\alpha, \beta)}{\partial \beta} \\ \dfrac{\partial h(\alpha, \beta)}{\partial \alpha} & \dfrac{\partial h(\alpha, \beta)}{\partial \beta} \end{vmatrix}, \qquad (6.43)$$

where the indicated partial derivatives are assumed to exist. Typically, the most difficult aspect of the joint PDF technique is in solving the simultaneous equations. The joint PDF technique can also be used to find the probability distribution for $z = g(x, y)$ from $f_{x,y}$ by introducing an auxiliary random variable $w = h(x, y)$ to find $f_{z,w}$, and then integrating to obtain the marginal PDF f_z.

6.6   PROBLEMS

1. Let random variable x be uniform between 0 and 2 with $z = \exp(x)$. Find F_z using the CDF technique.

2. Given

$$f_x(\alpha) = \begin{cases} 0.5(1+\alpha), & -1 < \alpha < 1 \\ 0, & \text{otherwise,} \end{cases}$$

and

$$z = \begin{cases} x - 1, & x < 0 \\ x + 1, & x > 0. \end{cases}$$

Use the CDF technique to find F_z.

3. Suppose random variable x has the CDF

$$F_x(\alpha) = \begin{cases} 0, & \alpha < 0 \\ \alpha^2, & 0 \leq \alpha < 1 \\ 1, & 1 \leq \alpha \end{cases}$$

and $z = \exp(-x)$. Using the CDF technique, find F_z.

76 ADVANCED PROBABILITY THEORY FOR BIOMEDICAL ENGINEERS

4. The PDF of random variable x is

$$f_x(\alpha) = \frac{1}{2} e^{-\frac{1}{2}(\alpha+2)} u(\alpha + 2).$$

Find F_z using the CDF technique when $z = |x|$.

5. Suppose random variable x has the PDF

$$f_x(\alpha) = \begin{cases} 2\alpha, & 0 < \alpha < 1 \\ 0, & \text{otherwise.} \end{cases}$$

Random variable z is defined by

$$z = \begin{cases} -1, & x \leq -1 \\ x, & -1 < x < 1 \\ 1, & x \geq 1. \end{cases}$$

Using the CDF method, determine F_z.

6. Random variable x represents the input to a half-wave rectifier and z represents the output, so that $z = u(x)$. Given that x is uniformly distributed between -2 and 2, find: (a) $E(z)$ using f_x, (b) F_z using the CDF method, (c) f_z, (d) $E(z)$ using f_z (compare with the answer to part a).

7. Random variable x represents the input to a full-wave rectifier and z represents the output, so that $z = |x|$. Given that x is uniformly distributed between -2 and 2, find: (a) $E(z)$ using f_x, (b) F_z using the CDF method, (c) f_z, (d) $E(z)$ using f_z (compare with the answer to part a).

8. Random variable x has the PDF $f_x(\alpha) = e^{-\alpha} u(\alpha)$. Find F_z for $z = x^2$ using the CDF method.

9. Given

$$f_x(\alpha) = \frac{a}{1+\alpha^2}$$

and

$$z = \begin{cases} -1, & x < -1 \\ x, & -1 \leq x \leq 2 \\ 2, & x > 2. \end{cases}$$

Determine: (a) a, (b) F_z.

10. Random variables x and z are the input and output of a quantizer. The relationship between them is defined by:

$$z = \begin{cases} 0, & x < 0.5 \\ 1, & 0.5 \leq x < 1.5 \\ 2, & 1.5 \leq x < 2.5 \\ 3, & 2.5 \leq x < 3.5 \\ 4, & x \geq 3.5. \end{cases}$$

Given that the input follows a Gaussian distribution with $x \sim G(2.25, 0.49)$, find f_z using the CDF method.

11. Random variable x has the PDF $f_x(\alpha) = e^{-\alpha}u(\alpha)$. With $z = 100 - 25x$, find: (a) F_z using the CDF technique, (b) F_z using the PDF technique.

12. Random variable x has the following PDF

$$f_x(\alpha) = \begin{cases} 4\alpha^3, & 0 < \alpha < 1 \\ 0, & \text{otherwise.} \end{cases}$$

Find the PDFs for the following random variables: (a) $z = x^3$, (b) $z = (x - 1/2)^2$, (c) $z = (x - 1/4)^2$.

13. Random variable x has the CDF

$$F_x(\alpha) = \begin{cases} 0, & \alpha < -1 \\ (\alpha^2 + 2\alpha + 1)/9, & -1 \leq \alpha < 2 \\ 1, & 2 \leq \alpha \end{cases}$$

and

$$z = \begin{cases} x, & x < -0.5 \\ 0, & -0.5 \leq x \leq 0 \\ x, & 0 < x. \end{cases}$$

Determine F_z.

14. Suppose

$$f_x(\alpha) = \begin{cases} (1 + \alpha^2)/6, & -1 < \alpha < 2 \\ 0, & \text{otherwise.} \end{cases}$$

Let $z = 1/x^2$. Use the CDF technique to determine F_z.

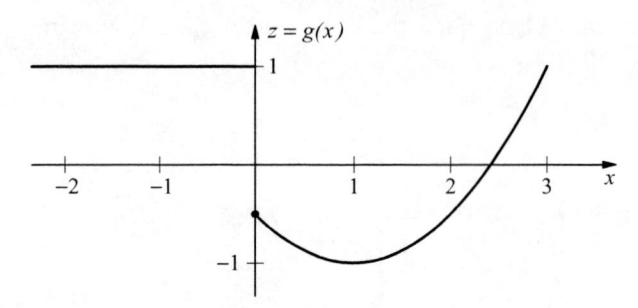

FIGURE 6.12: Plot for Problem 15.

15. Random variable x has the CDF

$$F_x(\alpha) = \begin{cases} 0, & \alpha < -1 \\ 0.25(\alpha + 1), & -1 \leq \alpha < 3 \\ 1, & 3 \leq \alpha. \end{cases}$$

Find the CDF F_z, with RV $z = g(x)$, and $g(x)$ shown in Figure 6.12. Assume that $g(x)$ is a second degree polynomial for $x \geq 0$.

16. The voltage x in Figure 6.13 is a random variable which is uniformly distributed from -1 to 2. Find the PDF f_z. Assume the diode is ideal.

17. The voltage x in Figure 6.14 is a Gaussian random variable with mean $\eta_x = 0$ and standard deviation $\sigma_x = 3$. Find the PDF f_z. Assume the diodes are ideal.

18. The voltage x in Figure 6.15 is a Gaussian random variable with mean $\eta_x = 1$ and standard deviation $\sigma_x = 1$. Find the PDF f_z. Assume the diode and the operational amplifier are ideal.

19. Random variable x is Gaussian with mean $\eta_x = 0$ and standard deviation $\sigma_x = 1$. With $z = g(x)$ shown in Figure 6.16, find the PDF f_z.

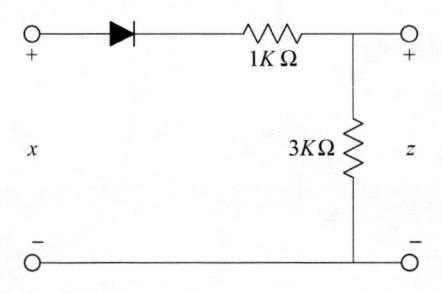

FIGURE 6.13: Circuit for Problem 16.

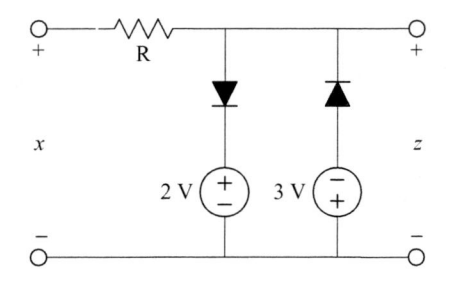

FIGURE 6.14: Circuit for Problem 17.

20. Random variable x has the following PDF

$$f_x(\alpha) = \begin{cases} \alpha + 0.5\delta(\alpha - 0.5), & 0 < \alpha < 1 \\ 0, & \text{otherwise.} \end{cases}$$

Find F_z if $z = x^2$.

21. Random variable x is uniform in the interval 0 to 12. Random variable $z = 4x + 2$. Find f_z using the PDF technique.

22. Find f_z if $z = 1/x^2$ and x is uniform on -1 to 2.

23. Random variable x has the PDF

$$f_x(\alpha) = \begin{cases} 2(\alpha + 1)/9, & -1 < \alpha < 2 \\ 0, & \text{otherwise.} \end{cases}$$

Find the PDF of $z = 2x^2$ using the PDF technique.

24. Let $z = \cos(x)$. Find f_z if:

(a) $f_x(\alpha) = \begin{cases} 1/\pi, & |\alpha| < \pi/2 \\ 0, & \text{otherwise.} \end{cases}$

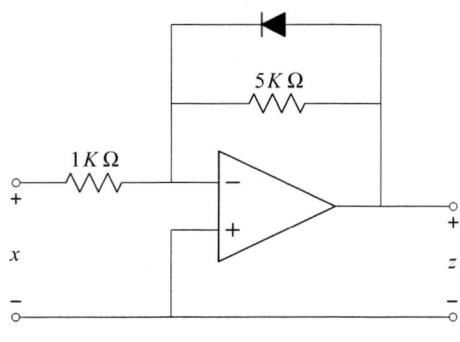

FIGURE 6.15: Circuit for Problem 18.

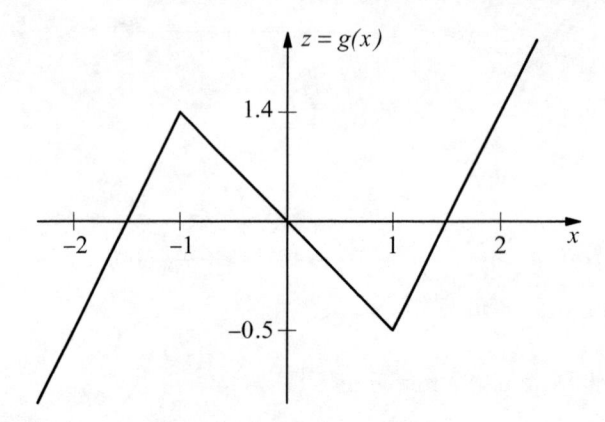

FIGURE 6.16: Transformation for Problem 19.

(b) $f_x(\alpha) = \begin{cases} 8\alpha/\pi^2, & 0 < \alpha < \pi/2 \\ 0, & \text{otherwise.} \end{cases}$

25. Given that x has the CDF

$$F_x(\alpha) = \begin{cases} 0, & \alpha < 0 \\ \alpha, & 0 \le \alpha < 1 \\ 1, & 1 \le \alpha. \end{cases}$$

Find the PDF of $z = -2\ln(x)$ using the PDF technique.

26. Random variable x has the PDF

$$f_x(\alpha) = \begin{cases} 2\alpha/9, & 0 < \alpha < 3 \\ 0, & \text{otherwise.} \end{cases}$$

Random variable $z = (x-1)^2$ and event $A = \{x : x \ge 1/2\}$. Find the PDF of random variable z, given event A.

27. Random variable x is uniform between -1 and 1. Random variable

$$z = \begin{cases} x^2, & x < 0 \\ x, & x \ge 0. \end{cases}$$

Using the PDF technique, find f_z.

28. A voltage v is a Gaussian random variable with $\eta_v = 0$ and $\sigma_v = 2$. Random variable $w = v^2/R$ represents the power dissipated in a resistor of $R\Omega$ with v volts across the resistor. Find (a) f_w, (b) $f_{w|A}$ if $A = \{v \ge 0\}$.

29. Random variable x has an exponential distribution with mean one. If $z = e^{-x}$, use the PDF technique to determine: (a) $f_{z|A}(\gamma|A)$ if $A = \{x : x > 2\}$, (b) $f_{z|B}(\gamma|B)$ if $B = \{z : z < 1/2\}$.

30. Find f_z if $z = 1/x$ and
$$f_x(\alpha) = \frac{1}{\pi(\alpha^2 + 1)}.$$

31. Given that random variable x has the PDF
$$f_x(\alpha) = \begin{cases} \alpha, & 0 < \alpha < 1 \\ 2 - \alpha, & 1 < \alpha < 2 \\ 0, & \text{otherwise.} \end{cases}$$
Using the PDF technique, find the PDF of $z = x^2$.

32. Suppose
$$f_x(\alpha) = \begin{cases} 2\alpha, & 0 < \alpha < 1 \\ 0, & \text{otherwise,} \end{cases}$$
and $z = 8x^3$. Determine f_z using the PDF technique.

33. Given
$$f_x(\alpha) = \begin{cases} 9\alpha^2, & 0 < \alpha < 0.5 \\ 3(1 - \alpha^2), & 0.5 < \alpha < 1 \\ 0, & \text{otherwise,} \end{cases}$$
and $z = -2\ln(x)$. Determine: (a) f_z, (b) F_z, (c) $E(z)$, (d) $E(z^2)$.

34. Using the PDF technique, find f_z if $z = |x|$ and x is a standard Gaussian random variable.

35. Suppose RV x has PDF $f_x(\alpha) = 0.5\alpha(u(\alpha) - u(\alpha - 2))$. Find a transformation g such that $z = g(x)$ has PDF
$$f_z(\gamma) = c\gamma^2(u(\gamma) - u(\gamma - 1)).$$

36. Let
$$f_x(\alpha) = \begin{cases} 0.75(1 - \alpha^2), & -1 < \alpha < 1 \\ 0, & \text{otherwise,} \end{cases}$$
and $z = x^2$. Determine f_z using the PDF technique.

37. Find f_z if $z = \sin(x)$ and
$$f_x(\alpha) = \begin{cases} 1/(2\pi), & 0 \le \alpha < 2\pi \\ 0, & \text{otherwise.} \end{cases}$$

38. Random variable x has the PDF
$$f_x(\alpha) = \begin{cases} 0.5, & -1 < \alpha < 0 \\ 0.5 - 0.25\alpha, & 0 < \alpha < 2 \\ 0, & \text{otherwise.} \end{cases}$$

(a) Find the transformation $z = g(x)$ so that
$$f_z(\gamma) = \begin{cases} 1 - 0.25\gamma, & 0 < \gamma < 1 \\ 0.5 - 0.25\gamma, & 1 < \gamma < 2 \\ 0, & \text{otherwise.} \end{cases}$$

(b) Determine f_z if $z = (2x + 2)u(x)$.

39. Let random variable x have the PDF
$$f_x(\alpha) = \begin{cases} 1/12, & -2 < \alpha < 1 \\ 1/4, & 1 < \alpha < 2; \end{cases}$$

in addition, $P(x = -2) = P(x = 2) = 0.25$. If $z = 1/x$, find f_z.

40. Random variable x has PDF
$$f_x(\alpha) = \frac{1}{4}\delta(\alpha + 1) + \frac{1}{4}\delta(\alpha) + (u(\alpha) - u(\alpha - 2)).$$

Random variable $z = g(x)$, with g shown in Figure 6.17. Find the PDF f_z.

41. Random variable x has PDF
$$f_x(\alpha) = \frac{\alpha^2}{3}(u(\alpha + 1) - u(\alpha - 2)).$$

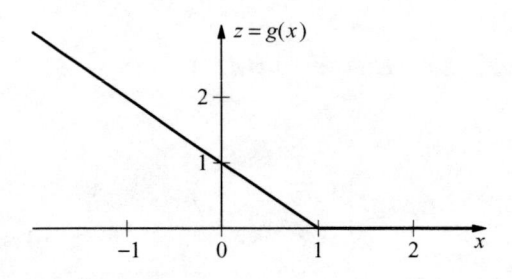

FIGURE 6.17: Transformation for Problem 40.

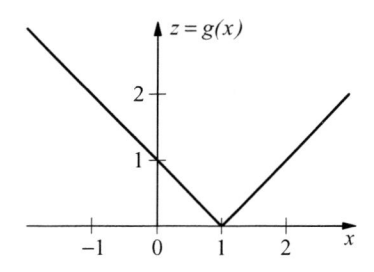

FIGURE 6.18: Transformation for Problem 41.

Random variable $z = g(x)$, with g shown in Figure 6.18. Use the PDF technique to find: (a) f_z, (b) $f_{z|A}$ with $A = \{x > 0\}$.

42. The PDF for random variable x is $f_x(\alpha) = e^{-\alpha}u(\alpha)$. With $z = e^{-x}$, determine: (a) $f_{z|A}(\gamma|A)$ where $A = \{x : x > 2\}$, (b) $f_{z|B}(\gamma|B)$ where $B = \{z : z < 1/2\}$.

43. The joint PDF of x and y is

$$f_{x,y}(\alpha, \beta) = \begin{cases} e^{-\alpha}, & 0 < \beta < \alpha \\ 0, & \text{otherwise.} \end{cases}$$

With $z = x + y$, write an expression(s) for $F_z(\gamma)$ (do not solve, just write the integral(s) necessary to find F_z.

44. If $z = x/y$, find F_z when x and y have the joint PDF

$$f_{x,y}(\alpha, \beta) = \begin{cases} 0.25\alpha, & 0 < \beta < \alpha < 1 \\ 0, & \text{otherwise.} \end{cases}$$

45. Resistors R_1 and R_2 have values r_1 and r_2 which are independent RVs uniformly distributed between $1\,\Omega$ and $2\,\Omega$. With r denoting the equivalent resistance of a series connection of R_1 and R_2, find the PDF f_r using convolution.

46. Resistors R_1 and R_2 have values r_1 and r_2 which are independent RVs uniformly distributed between $1\,\Omega$ and $2\,\Omega$. With g denoting the equivalent conductance of a parallel connection of R_1 and R_2, find the PDF f_g using convolution.

47. Suppose the voltage v across a resistor is a random variable with PDF

$$f_v(\alpha) = \begin{cases} 6\alpha(1-\alpha), & 0 < \alpha < 1 \\ 0, & \text{otherwise,} \end{cases}$$

and that resistance r is a random variable with PDF

$$f_r(\beta) = \begin{cases} 1/12, & 94 < \beta < 106 \\ 0, & \text{otherwise.} \end{cases}$$

Moreover, suppose that v and r are independent random variables. Find the PDF for power, $p = v^2/r$.

48. The joint PDF for random variables x and y is

$$f_{x,y}(\alpha, \beta) = \begin{cases} \alpha + \beta, & 0 < \alpha < 1, 0 < \beta < 1 \\ 0, & \text{otherwise.} \end{cases}$$

Let $z = 2x + y$ and $w = x + 2y$. Find $f_{z,w}$.

49. The joint PDF for random variables x and y is

$$f_{x,y}(\alpha, \beta) = \begin{cases} 4\alpha\beta, & 0 < \alpha < 1, 0 < \beta < 1 \\ 0, & \text{otherwise.} \end{cases}$$

Let $z = x^2$ and $w = xy$. Find: (a) $f_{z,w}$, (b) f_z.

50. The joint PDF for random variables x and y is

$$f_{x,y}(\alpha, \beta) = \begin{cases} 3(\alpha^2 + \beta^2), & 0 < \beta < \alpha < 1 \\ 0, & \text{otherwise.} \end{cases}$$

Find the joint PDF for random variables $z = x + y$ and $w = x - y$.

51. The joint PDF for random variables x and y is

$$f_{x,y}(\alpha, \beta) = \begin{cases} 0.5\beta e^{-\alpha}, & 0 < \alpha, 0 < \beta < 2 \\ 0, & \text{otherwise.} \end{cases}$$

With $z = y/x$, find f_z.

52. The joint PDF for random variables x and y is

$$f_{x,y}(\alpha, \beta) = \begin{cases} 8\alpha\beta, & 0 < \alpha^2 + \beta^2 < 1, 0 < \alpha, 0 < \beta \\ 0, & \text{otherwise.} \end{cases}$$

Let $A = \{(x, y) : x > y\}$, $z = x$ and $w = x^2 + y^2$. Find: (a) $f_{z,w|A}$, (b) $f_{z|A}$.

53. The joint PDF for random variables x and y is

$$f_{x,y}(\alpha, \beta) = \begin{cases} 1/\alpha, & 0 < \beta < \alpha < 1 \\ 0, & \text{otherwise.} \end{cases}$$

Let $z = x/y$ and $w = y$. Find $f_{z,w}$.

54. The joint PDF for random variables x and y is

$$f_{x,y}(\alpha, \beta) = \begin{cases} \alpha \sin(\beta), & 0 < \alpha < 1, 0 < \beta < \pi \\ 0, & \text{otherwise.} \end{cases}$$

Let $z = x^2$ and $w = \cos(y)$. Find $f_{z,w}$.

55. The joint PDF for random variables x and y is

$$f_{x,y}(\alpha, \beta) = \begin{cases} 12\alpha\beta(1-\alpha), & 0 < \alpha < 1, 0 < \beta < 1 \\ 0, & \text{otherwise.} \end{cases}$$

Let $z = x^2 y$. Find f_z.

56. The joint PDF for random variables x and y is

$$f_{x,y}(\alpha, \beta) = \begin{cases} e^{-\alpha-\beta}, & 0 < \alpha, 0 < \beta \\ 0, & \text{otherwise.} \end{cases}$$

Let $z = x + y$ and $w = x/(x+y)$. Find: (a) $f_{z,w}$, (b) f_z.

57. The joint PDF for random variables x and y is

$$f_{x,y}(\alpha, \beta) = \begin{cases} 0.25(\alpha + \beta), & |\alpha| < 1, |\beta| < 1 \\ 0, & \text{otherwise.} \end{cases}$$

Let $z = xy$ and $w = y/x$. Find $f_{z,w}$ using the joint CDF technique.

APPENDIX A

Distribution Tables

TABLE A.1: Bernoulli CDF for $n = 5$ and $n = 10$

$n = 5$

p	k	+0	+1	+2	+3	+4
0.05	0	0.773781	0.977408	0.998842	0.999970	1.000000
0.1	0	0.590490	0.918540	0.991440	0.999540	0.999990
0.15	0	0.443705	0.835210	0.973388	0.997773	0.999924
0.2	0	0.327680	0.737280	0.942080	0.993280	0.999680
0.25	0	0.237305	0.632813	0.896484	0.984375	0.999023
0.3	0	0.168070	0.528220	0.836920	0.969220	0.997570
0.35	0	0.116029	0.428415	0.764831	0.945978	0.994748
0.4	0	0.077760	0.336960	0.682560	0.912960	0.989760
0.45	0	0.050328	0.256218	0.593127	0.868780	0.981547
0.5	0	0.031250	0.187500	0.500000	0.812500	0.968750

$n = 10$

p	k	+0	+1	+2	+3	+4
0.05	0	0.598737	0.913862	0.988496	0.998971	0.999936
	5	0.999997	1.000000	1.000000	1.000000	1.000000
0.1	0	0.348678	0.736099	0.929809	0.987205	0.998365
	5	0.999853	0.999991	1.000000	1.000000	1.000000
0.15	0	0.196874	0.544300	0.820197	0.950030	0.990126
	5	0.998617	0.999865	0.999991	1.000000	1.000000

(*Continued*)

TABLE A.1: Bernoulli CDF for $n = 5$ and $n = 10$ (Continued)

				$n = 10$		
p	k	+0	+1	+2	+3	+4
0.2	0	0.107374	0.375810	0.677800	0.879126	0.967206
	5	0.993631	0.999136	0.999922	0.999996	1.000000
0.25	0	0.056314	0.244025	0.525593	0.775875	0.921873
	5	0.980272	0.996494	0.999584	0.999970	0.999999
0.3	0	0.028248	0.149308	0.382783	0.649611	0.849732
	5	0.952651	0.989408	0.998410	0.999856	0.999994
0.35	0	0.013463	0.085954	0.261607	0.513827	0.751495
	5	0.905066	0.973976	0.995179	0.999460	0.999972
0.4	0	0.006047	0.046357	0.167290	0.382281	0.633103
	5	0.833761	0.945238	0.987705	0.998322	0.999895
0.45	0	0.002533	0.023257	0.099560	0.266038	0.504405
	5	0.738437	0.898005	0.972608	0.995498	0.999659
0.5	0	0.000977	0.010742	0.054688	0.171875	0.376953
	5	0.623047	0.828125	0.945313	0.989258	0.999023

TABLE A.2: Bernoulli CDF for $n = 15$

				$n = 15$		
p	k	+0	+1	+2	+3	+4
0.05	0	0.463291	0.829047	0.963800	0.994533	0.999385
	5	0.999947	0.999996	1.000000	1.000000	1.000000
	10	1.000000	1.000000	1.000000	1.000000	1.000000
0.1	0	0.205891	0.549043	0.815939	0.944444	0.987280
	5	0.997750	0.999689	0.999966	0.999997	1.000000
	10	1.000000	1.000000	1.000000	1.000000	1.000000

TABLE A.2: Bernoulli CDF for $n = 15$ *(Continued)*

p	k	+0	+1	+2	+3	+4
0.15	0	0.087354	0.318586	0.604225	0.822655	0.938295
	5	0.983190	0.996394	0.999390	0.999919	0.999992
	10	0.999999	1.000000	1.000000	1.000000	1.000000
0.2	0	0.035184	0.167126	0.398023	0.648162	0.835766
	5	0.938949	0.981941	0.995760	0.999215	0.999887
	10	0.999988	0.999999	1.000000	1.000000	1.000000
0.25	0	0.013363	0.080181	0.236088	0.461287	0.686486
	5	0.851632	0.943380	0.982700	0.995807	0.999205
	10	0.999885	0.999988	0.999999	1.000000	1.000000
0.3	0	0.004748	0.035268	0.126828	0.296868	0.515491
	5	0.721621	0.868857	0.949987	0.984757	0.996347
	10	0.999328	0.999908	0.999991	1.000000	1.000000
0.35	0	0.001562	0.014179	0.061734	0.172696	0.351943
	5	0.564282	0.754842	0.886769	0.957806	0.987557
	10	0.997169	0.999521	0.999943	0.999996	1.000000
0.4	0	0.000470	0.005172	0.027114	0.090502	0.217278
	5	0.403216	0.609813	0.786897	0.904953	0.966167
	10	0.990652	0.998072	0.999721	0.999975	0.999999
0.45	0	0.000127	0.001692	0.010652	0.042421	0.120399
	5	0.260760	0.452160	0.653504	0.818240	0.923071
	10	0.974534	0.993673	0.998893	0.999879	0.999994
0.5	0	0.000031	0.000488	0.003693	0.017578	0.059235
	5	0.150879	0.303619	0.500000	0.696381	0.849121
	10	0.940765	0.982422	0.996307	0.999512	0.999969

TABLE A.3: Bernoulli CDF for $n = 20$

		\multicolumn{5}{c	}{$n = 20$}
p	k	+0	+1	+2	+3	+4
0.05	0	0.358486	0.735840	0.924516	0.984098	0.997426
	5	0.999671	0.999966	0.999997	1.000000	1.000000
	10	1.000000	1.000000	1.000000	1.000000	1.000000
	15	1.000000	1.000000	1.000000	1.000000	1.000000
0.1	0	0.121577	0.391747	0.676927	0.867047	0.956825
	5	0.988747	0.997614	0.999584	0.999940	0.999993
	10	0.999999	1.000000	1.000000	1.000000	1.000000
	15	1.000000	1.000000	1.000000	1.000000	1.000000
0.15	0	0.038760	0.175558	0.404896	0.647725	0.829847
	5	0.932692	0.978065	0.994079	0.998671	0.999752
	10	0.999961	0.999995	0.999999	1.000000	1.000000
	15	1.000000	1.000000	1.000000	1.000000	1.000000
0.2	0	0.011529	0.069175	0.206085	0.411449	0.629648
	5	0.804208	0.913307	0.967857	0.990018	0.997405
	10	0.999437	0.999898	0.999985	0.999998	1.000000
	15	1.000000	1.000000	1.000000	1.000000	1.000000
0.25	0	0.003171	0.024313	0.091260	0.225156	0.414842
	5	0.617173	0.785782	0.898188	0.959075	0.986136
	10	0.996058	0.999065	0.999816	0.999970	0.999996
	15	1.000000	1.000000	1.000000	1.000000	1.000000
0.3	0	0.000798	0.007637	0.035483	0.107087	0.237508
	5	0.416371	0.608010	0.772272	0.886669	0.952038
	10	0.982855	0.994862	0.998721	0.999739	0.999957
	15	0.999994	0.999999	1.000000	1.000000	1.000000
0.35	0	0.000181	0.002133	0.012118	0.044376	0.118197
	5	0.245396	0.416625	0.601027	0.762378	0.878219
	10	0.946833	0.980421	0.993985	0.998479	0.999689
	15	0.999950	0.999994	0.999999	1.000000	1.000000

TABLE A.3: Bernoulli CDF for $n = 20$ (Continued)

$n = 20$

p	k	+0	+1	+2	+3	+4
0.4	0	0.000037	0.000524	0.003611	0.015961	0.050952
	5	0.125599	0.250011	0.415893	0.595599	0.755337
	10	0.872479	0.943474	0.978971	0.993534	0.998388
	15	0.999683	0.999953	0.999995	1.000000	1.000000
0.45	0	0.000006	0.000111	0.000927	0.004933	0.018863
	5	0.055334	0.129934	0.252006	0.414306	0.591361
	10	0.750711	0.869235	0.941966	0.978586	0.993566
	15	0.998469	0.999723	0.999964	0.999997	1.000000
0.5	0	0.000001	0.000020	0.000201	0.001288	0.005909
	5	0.020695	0.057659	0.131588	0.251722	0.411901
	10	0.588099	0.748278	0.868412	0.942341	0.979305
	15	0.994091	0.998712	0.999799	0.999980	0.999999

TABLE A.4: Poisson CDF for $\lambda = 0.1, 0.2, \ldots, 1, 1.5, 2, \ldots, 4.5$

λ	k	+0	+1	+2	+3	+4
0.1	0	0.904837	0.995321	0.999845	0.999996	1.000000
0.2	0	0.818731	0.982477	0.998852	0.999943	0.999998
0.3	0	0.740818	0.963064	0.996400	0.999734	0.999984
0.4	0	0.670320	0.938448	0.992074	0.999224	0.999939
0.5	0	0.606531	0.909796	0.985612	0.998248	0.999828
	5	0.999986	0.999999	1.000000	1.000000	1.000000
0.6	0	0.548812	0.878099	0.976885	0.996642	0.999605
	5	0.999961	0.999997	1.000000	1.000000	1.000000
0.7	0	0.496585	0.844195	0.965858	0.994247	0.999214
	5	0.999910	0.999991	0.999999	1.000000	1.000000

(*Continued*)

TABLE A.4: Poisson CDF for $\lambda = 0.1, 0.2, \ldots, 1, 1.5, 2, \ldots, 4.5$ *(Continued)*

λ	k	+0	+1	+2	+3	+4
0.8	0	0.449329	0.808792	0.952577	0.990920	0.998589
	5	0.999816	0.999979	0.999998	1.000000	1.000000
0.9	0	0.406570	0.772482	0.937143	0.986541	0.997656
	5	0.999656	0.999957	0.999995	1.000000	1.000000
1	0	0.367879	0.735759	0.919699	0.981012	0.996340
	5	0.999406	0.999917	0.999990	0.999999	1.000000
1.5	0	0.223130	0.557825	0.808847	0.934358	0.981424
	5	0.995544	0.999074	0.999830	0.999972	0.999996
2	0	0.135335	0.406006	0.676676	0.857123	0.947347
	5	0.983436	0.995466	0.998903	0.999763	0.999954
2.5	0	0.082085	0.287297	0.543813	0.757576	0.891178
	5	0.957979	0.985813	0.995753	0.998860	0.999723
	10	0.999938	0.999987	0.999998	1.000000	1.000000
3	0	0.049787	0.199148	0.423190	0.647232	0.815263
	5	0.916082	0.966491	0.988095	0.996197	0.998897
	10	0.999708	0.999929	0.999984	0.999997	0.999999
3.5	0	0.030197	0.135888	0.320847	0.536633	0.725445
	5	0.857614	0.934712	0.973261	0.990126	0.996685
	10	0.998981	0.999711	0.999924	0.999981	0.999996
4	0	0.018316	0.091578	0.238103	0.433470	0.628837
	5	0.785130	0.889326	0.948866	0.978637	0.991868
	10	0.997160	0.999085	0.999726	0.999924	0.999980
4.5	0	0.011109	0.061099	0.173578	0.342296	0.532104
	5	0.702930	0.831051	0.913414	0.959743	0.982907
	10	0.993331	0.997596	0.999195	0.999748	0.999926
	15	0.999980	0.999995	0.999999	1.000000	1.000000

TABLE A.5: Poisson CDF for $\lambda = 5, 5.5, \ldots, 8.5$

λ	k	+0	+1	+2	+3	+4
5	0	0.006738	0.040428	0.124652	0.265026	0.440493
	5	0.615961	0.762183	0.866628	0.931906	0.968172
	10	0.986305	0.994547	0.997981	0.999302	0.999774
	15	0.999931	0.999980	0.999995	0.999999	1.000000
5.5	0	0.004087	0.026564	0.088376	0.201699	0.357518
	5	0.528919	0.686036	0.809485	0.894357	0.946223
	10	0.974749	0.989012	0.995549	0.998315	0.999401
	15	0.999800	0.999937	0.999981	0.999995	0.999999
6	0	0.002479	0.017351	0.061969	0.151204	0.285057
	5	0.445680	0.606303	0.743980	0.847238	0.916076
	10	0.957379	0.979908	0.991173	0.996372	0.998600
	15	0.999491	0.999825	0.999943	0.999982	0.999995
6.5	0	0.001503	0.011276	0.043036	0.111850	0.223672
	5	0.369041	0.526524	0.672758	0.791573	0.877384
	10	0.933161	0.966120	0.983973	0.992900	0.997044
	15	0.998840	0.999570	0.999849	0.999949	0.999984
7	0	0.000912	0.007295	0.029636	0.081765	0.172992
	5	0.300708	0.449711	0.598714	0.729091	0.830496
	10	0.901479	0.946650	0.973000	0.987189	0.994283
	15	0.997593	0.999042	0.999638	0.999870	0.999956
7.5	0	0.000553	0.004701	0.020257	0.059145	0.132062
	5	0.241436	0.378155	0.524639	0.661967	0.776408
	10	0.862238	0.920759	0.957334	0.978435	0.989740
	15	0.995392	0.998041	0.999210	0.999697	0.999889
	20	0.999961	0.999987	0.999996	0.999999	1.000000

(*Continued*)

TABLE A.5: Poisson CDF for $\lambda = 5, 5.5, \ldots, 8.5$ (Continued)

λ	k	+0	+1	+2	+3	+4
8	0	0.000335	0.003019	0.013754	0.042380	0.099632
	5	0.191236	0.313374	0.452961	0.592547	0.716624
	10	0.815886	0.888076	0.936203	0.965819	0.982743
	15	0.991769	0.996282	0.998406	0.999350	0.999747
	20	0.999906	0.999967	0.999989	0.999996	0.999999
8.5	0	0.000203	0.001933	0.009283	0.030109	0.074364
	5	0.149597	0.256178	0.385597	0.523105	0.652974
	10	0.763362	0.848662	0.909083	0.948589	0.972575
	15	0.986167	0.993387	0.996998	0.998703	0.999465
	20	0.999789	0.999921	0.999971	0.999990	0.999997

TABLE A.6: Poisson CDF for $\lambda = 9, 9.5, 10, 11, 12, 13$

λ	k	+0	+1	+2	+3	+4
9	0	0.000123	0.001234	0.006232	0.021226	0.054964
	5	0.115691	0.206781	0.323897	0.455653	0.587408
	10	0.705988	0.803008	0.875773	0.926149	0.958534
	15	0.977964	0.988894	0.994680	0.997574	0.998944
	20	0.999561	0.999825	0.999933	0.999975	0.999991
9.5	0	0.000075	0.000786	0.004164	0.014860	0.040263
	5	0.088528	0.164949	0.268663	0.391824	0.521826
	10	0.645328	0.751990	0.836430	0.898136	0.940008
	15	0.966527	0.982273	0.991072	0.995716	0.998038
	20	0.999141	0.999639	0.999855	0.999944	0.999979
10	0	0.000045	0.000499	0.002769	0.010336	0.029253
	5	0.067086	0.130141	0.220221	0.332820	0.457930
	10	0.583040	0.696776	0.791556	0.864464	0.916542

TABLE A.6: Poisson CDF for λ = 9, 9.5, 10, 11, 12, 13 *(Continued)*

λ	k	+0	+1	+2	+3	+4
	15	0.951260	0.972958	0.985722	0.992813	0.996546
	20	0.998412	0.999300	0.999704	0.999880	0.999953
11	0	0.000017	0.000200	0.001211	0.004916	0.015105
	5	0.037520	0.078614	0.143192	0.231985	0.340511
	10	0.459889	0.579267	0.688697	0.781291	0.854044
	15	0.907396	0.944076	0.967809	0.982313	0.990711
	20	0.995329	0.997748	0.998958	0.999536	0.999801
	25	0.999918	0.999967	0.999987	0.999995	0.999998
12	0	0.000006	0.000080	0.000522	0.002292	0.007600
	5	0.020341	0.045822	0.089505	0.155028	0.242392
	10	0.347229	0.461597	0.575965	0.681536	0.772025
	15	0.844416	0.898709	0.937034	0.962584	0.978720
	20	0.988402	0.993935	0.996953	0.998527	0.999314
	25	0.999692	0.999867	0.999944	0.999977	0.999991
13	0	0.000002	0.000032	0.000223	0.001050	0.003740
	5	0.010734	0.025887	0.054028	0.099758	0.165812
	10	0.251682	0.353165	0.463105	0.573045	0.675132
	15	0.763607	0.835493	0.890465	0.930167	0.957331
	20	0.974988	0.985919	0.992378	0.996028	0.998006
	25	0.999034	0.999548	0.999796	0.999911	0.999962

TABLE A.7: Poisson CDF for λ = 14, 15, 16, 17, 18

λ	k	+0	+1	+2	+3	+4
14	0	0.000001	0.000012	0.000094	0.000474	0.001805
	5	0.005532	0.014228	0.031620	0.062055	0.109399
	10	0.175681	0.260040	0.358458	0.464448	0.570437

(Continued)

TABLE A.7: Poisson CDF for $\lambda = 14, 15, 16, 17, 18$ *(Continued)*

λ	k	+0	+1	+2	+3	+4
	15	0.669360	0.755918	0.827201	0.882643	0.923495
	20	0.952092	0.971156	0.983288	0.990672	0.994980
	25	0.997392	0.998691	0.999365	0.999702	0.999864
	30	0.999940	0.999974	0.999989	0.999996	0.999998
15	0	0.000000	0.000005	0.000039	0.000211	0.000857
	5	0.002792	0.007632	0.018002	0.037446	0.069854
	10	0.118464	0.184752	0.267611	0.363218	0.465654
	15	0.568090	0.664123	0.748859	0.819472	0.875219
	20	0.917029	0.946894	0.967256	0.980535	0.988835
	25	0.993815	0.996688	0.998284	0.999139	0.999582
	30	0.999803	0.999910	0.999960	0.999983	0.999993
16	0	0.000000	0.000002	0.000016	0.000093	0.000400
	5	0.001384	0.004006	0.010000	0.021987	0.043298
	10	0.077396	0.126993	0.193122	0.274511	0.367527
	15	0.466745	0.565962	0.659344	0.742349	0.812249
	20	0.868168	0.910773	0.941759	0.963314	0.977685
	25	0.986881	0.992541	0.995895	0.997811	0.998869
	30	0.999433	0.999724	0.999869	0.999940	0.999973
17	0	0.000000	0.000001	0.000007	0.000041	0.000185
	5	0.000675	0.002062	0.005433	0.012596	0.026125
	10	0.049124	0.084669	0.135024	0.200873	0.280833
	15	0.371454	0.467738	0.564023	0.654958	0.736322
	20	0.805481	0.861466	0.904728	0.936704	0.959354
	25	0.974755	0.984826	0.991166	0.995016	0.997273
	30	0.998552	0.999253	0.999626	0.999817	0.999913

TABLE A.7: Poisson CDF for λ = 14, 15, 16, 17, 18 *(Continued)*

λ	k	+0	+1	+2	+3	+4
18	0	0.000000	0.000000	0.000003	0.000018	0.000084
	5	0.000324	0.001043	0.002893	0.007056	0.015381
	10	0.030366	0.054887	0.091669	0.142598	0.208077
	15	0.286653	0.375050	0.468648	0.562245	0.650916
	20	0.730720	0.799124	0.855090	0.898890	0.931740
	25	0.955392	0.971766	0.982682	0.989700	0.994056
	30	0.996669	0.998187	0.999040	0.999506	0.999752

TABLE A.8: Marcum's Q function for $\alpha = 0, 0.01, \ldots, 1.99$

α	+0.00	+0.01	+0.02	+0.03	+0.04
0.00	0.500000	0.496011	0.492022	0.488033	0.484046
0.05	0.480061	0.476078	0.472097	0.468119	0.464144
0.10	0.460172	0.456205	0.452242	0.448283	0.444330
0.15	0.440382	0.436441	0.432505	0.428576	0.424655
0.20	0.420740	0.416834	0.412936	0.409046	0.405165
0.25	0.401294	0.397432	0.393580	0.389739	0.385908
0.30	0.382089	0.378281	0.374484	0.370700	0.366928
0.35	0.363169	0.359424	0.355691	0.351973	0.348268
0.40	0.344578	0.340903	0.337243	0.333598	0.329969
0.45	0.326355	0.322758	0.319178	0.315614	0.312067
0.50	0.308538	0.305026	0.301532	0.298056	0.294598
0.55	0.291160	0.287740	0.284339	0.280957	0.277595
0.60	0.274253	0.270931	0.267629	0.264347	0.261086
0.65	0.257846	0.254627	0.251429	0.248252	0.245097

(Continued)

TABLE A.8: Marcum's Q function for $\alpha = 0, 0.01, \ldots, 1.99$ *(Continued)*

α	+0.00	+0.01	+0.02	+0.03	+0.04
0.70	0.241964	0.238852	0.235762	0.232695	0.229650
0.75	0.226627	0.223627	0.220650	0.217695	0.214764
0.80	0.211855	0.208970	0.206108	0.203269	0.200454
0.85	0.197662	0.194894	0.192150	0.189430	0.186733
0.90	0.184060	0.181411	0.178786	0.176186	0.173609
0.95	0.171056	0.168528	0.166023	0.163543	0.161087
1.00	0.158655	0.156248	0.153864	0.151505	0.149170
1.05	0.146859	0.144572	0.142310	0.140071	0.137857
1.10	0.135666	0.133500	0.131357	0.129238	0.127143
1.15	0.125072	0.123024	0.121001	0.119000	0.117023
1.20	0.115070	0.113140	0.111233	0.109349	0.107488
1.25	0.105650	0.103835	0.102042	0.100273	0.098525
1.30	0.096801	0.095098	0.093418	0.091759	0.090123
1.35	0.088508	0.086915	0.085344	0.083793	0.082264
1.40	0.080757	0.079270	0.077804	0.076359	0.074934
1.45	0.073529	0.072145	0.070781	0.069437	0.068112
1.50	0.066807	0.065522	0.064256	0.063008	0.061780
1.55	0.060571	0.059380	0.058208	0.057053	0.055917
1.60	0.054799	0.053699	0.052616	0.051551	0.050503
1.65	0.049471	0.048457	0.047460	0.046479	0.045514
1.70	0.044565	0.043633	0.042716	0.041815	0.040929
1.75	0.040059	0.039204	0.038364	0.037538	0.036727
1.80	0.035930	0.035148	0.034379	0.033625	0.032884
1.85	0.032157	0.031443	0.030742	0.030054	0.029379
1.90	0.028716	0.028067	0.027429	0.026803	0.026190
1.95	0.025588	0.024998	0.024419	0.023852	0.023295

TABLE A.9: Marcum's Q function for $\alpha = 3, 3.01, \ldots, 3.99$

α	+0.00	+0.01	+0.02	+0.03	+0.04
2.00	0.022750	0.022216	0.021692	0.021178	0.020675
2.05	0.020182	0.019699	0.019226	0.018763	0.018309
2.10	0.017864	0.017429	0.017003	0.016586	0.016177
2.15	0.015778	0.015386	0.015003	0.014629	0.014262
2.20	0.013903	0.013553	0.013209	0.012874	0.012545
2.25	0.012224	0.011911	0.011604	0.011304	0.011011
2.30	0.010724	0.010444	0.010170	0.009903	0.009642
2.35	0.009387	0.009137	0.008894	0.008656	0.008424
2.40	0.008198	0.007976	0.007760	0.007549	0.007344
2.45	0.007143	0.006947	0.006756	0.006569	0.006387
2.50	0.006210	0.006037	0.005868	0.005703	0.005543
2.55	0.005386	0.005234	0.005085	0.004940	0.004799
2.60	0.004661	0.004527	0.004397	0.004269	0.004145
2.65	0.004025	0.003907	0.003793	0.003681	0.003573
2.70	0.003467	0.003364	0.003264	0.003167	0.003072
2.75	0.002980	0.002890	0.002803	0.002718	0.002635
2.80	0.002555	0.002477	0.002401	0.002327	0.002256
2.85	0.002186	0.002118	0.002052	0.001988	0.001926
2.90	0.001866	0.001807	0.001750	0.001695	0.001641
2.95	0.001589	0.001538	0.001489	0.001441	0.001395
3.00	0.001350	0.001306	0.001264	0.001223	0.001183
3.05	0.001144	0.001107	0.001070	0.001035	0.001001
3.10	0.000968	0.000936	0.000904	0.000874	0.000845
3.15	0.000816	0.000789	0.000762	0.000736	0.000711
3.20	0.000687	0.000664	0.000641	0.000619	0.000598
3.25	0.000577	0.000557	0.000538	0.000519	0.000501
3.30	0.000483	0.000467	0.000450	0.000434	0.000419

(*Continued*)

TABLE A.9: Marcum's Q function for $\alpha = 3, 3.01, \ldots, 3.99$ *(Continued)*

α	+0.00	+0.01	+0.02	+0.03	+0.04
3.35	0.000404	0.000390	0.000376	0.000362	0.000350
3.40	0.000337	0.000325	0.000313	0.000302	0.000291
3.45	0.000280	0.000270	0.000260	0.000251	0.000242
3.50	0.000233	0.000224	0.000216	0.000208	0.000200
3.55	0.000193	0.000185	0.000179	0.000172	0.000165
3.60	0.000159	0.000153	0.000147	0.000142	0.000136
3.65	0.000131	0.000126	0.000121	0.000117	0.000112
3.70	0.000108	0.000104	0.000100	0.000096	0.000092
3.75	0.000088	0.000085	0.000082	0.000078	0.000075
3.80	0.000072	0.000070	0.000067	0.000064	0.000062
3.85	0.000059	0.000057	0.000054	0.000052	0.000050
3.90	0.000048	0.000046	0.000044	0.000042	0.000041
3.95	0.000039	0.000037	0.000036	0.000034	0.000033